"I absolutely loved *Chocolate Yoga*. Whenever I'm feeling overloaded with commitments and chores, Margaret Chester's common-sense, yet comforting suggestions bring me instant peace. I can honestly say this book changed my life."

~ Susan Colleen Browne,
author of *Little Farm in the Foothills*

"For years, as a senior, I've taken many yoga classes and health sessions, but I found it difficult to continue on my own. Now, I feel I have Margaret Chester and *Chocolate Yoga* right in my home! It's the way she personally speaks to you in her special caring way, and almost predicts what your pitfalls will be. I hope she'll continue to write more; in the meantime, I'm inhaling, pausing, and exhaling…"

~ Marilyn Alper, Honolulu, HI

"I find my *Chocolate Yoga* several times a day while standing in front of my refrigerator. I no longer bother to open the door. Instead I stand quietly and slowly take five deep breaths. I am then ready to walk away, usually singing or humming, 'I got along without you before I met you, gonna get along without you now.' I feel so victorious. *Chocolate Yoga* is definitely my favorite snack."

~ Shirley B.

"This book is a life saver. I started a new job about the time that I started reading *Chocolate Yoga*. The job is stressful to say the least. Taking a moment every couple of hours to stop and breathe and do an internal life has made all the difference in the world."

~ B.A. Mayler, Bellingham, WA

"While doing the layout and design of this book I found the concepts and suggestions to be invaluable. I used the *Chocolate Yoga* breathing techniques to stay calm during biopsies and surgery. I'm sure this book helped me with my swift recovery."

~ Kate Weisel, Bellingham, WA

"This slim tome is filled with inspiring passages and techniques of how we can withhold snippets of our own days—just for ourselves. Margaret names these blessed moments "chocolate." She uses chocolate as a metaphor for those moments in time that nourish the soul. A few moments here, a few moments there when we are mindful of our breathing will make a difference. Exhale. Inhale. Breathe. These few moments a day of me nurturing me was making a difference."

~ Chanticleer Book Reviews & Media

"*Chocolate Yoga* is filled with inspiring passages and techniques, trail-blazing an entirely different approach to stress and weight management. It describes a way of life, brought to us in a reader-friendly, body-friendly guide to the basics of yoga. Not just mechanical poses or asanas, but a more mindful, well-rounded approach to health and life."

~ Matt McErlean

"As a women's health educator and coach I have been practicing yoga since I was a young girl and I am always seeking new ways to educate women to the value of a daily practice of yoga. *Chocolate Yoga* has beautifully captured the essence of yoga while inviting the reader to embark on the journey through a simple and joyful approach. Author Margaret Chester embraces the "art of living" providing tools for dealing with the challenges of life. Her words are uplifting and a sweet companion to every day. If you have never done yoga this is a great book to get you on the path and if you are a life-long student of yoga you will find joy in this new approach."

~ Wendy Mitchell, MA, CPC

Chocolate Yoga

A System of Yoga Techniques for Stress and Weight Management That Will Nurture Your Body, Mind and Spirit

Margaret Chester, MPH, RYT

Chocolate Yoga
A System of Yoga Techniques for Stress and Weight Management That
Will Nurture Your Body, Mind and Spirit.

First edition, 2011; revised, second printing

ISBN: 978-0-9831882-0-9
ebook ISBN: 978-0-9831882-1-6

Library of Congress Control Number: 2011929363

Printed in the United States of America

Book design, typography and ebook preparation by
Kathleen R. Weisel. (www.weiselcreative.com)

Dedication

This book is dedicated with loving kindness to all of us who struggle on a daily basis, to live and love the life that we were meant to live.

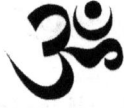

A sincere thank you to my family, friends, coworkers, neighbors, students and teachers, who have supported me throughout my life. And to everyone who has shared their ideas on how they use yoga techniques to manage their stress and weight issues.

Namaste.

A Brief Note Before We Begin

This is not a technical, scientific, or a scholarly treatise on yoga, stress, or weight management. It is my interpretation of a yoga, stress, and weight management system that works for me. Please consult a licensed health care practitioner for professional medical advice before making any changes in your routine.

Disclaimers

This publication contains the opinions and ideas of its author. It is intended to provide helpful and informative material on the subject matter covered. It is sold with the understanding that the author and publisher are not engaged in rendering professional services in the book. If the reader requires personal assistance or advice, a competent professional should be consulted.

The author and publisher specifically disclaim any responsibility for any liability, loss, injury or damage, personal or otherwise, incurred as a consequence, directly or indirectly, of the use and application of any information contained in this book.

- If you have any major health issues, please consult a licensed health care practitioner before you begin this program. You are responsible for setting limits for yourself at all times.
- This is NOT a proven medical science program. It is an experiential system that may or may not work for you. Please take your life seriously and continue to look for your answers.
- I am not a dietitian, nutritionist, or a physician. I will not tell you what to eat and what not to eat. You know what foods work for you. I am just awakening your personal powers to help you connect with your true self.
- Under no circumstances ignore any symptoms that may require a diagnosis, treatment, and active care under a licensed health care practitioner.
- Please acknowledge that we are all part of the problem and the solution—then have the courage to find your (own true) answer.

Contents

Visit

www.ChocolateYoga.com

**for more suggestions, updates, instructions
and guidance on using yoga techniques
to manage your stress and weight issues.**

Foreword

I have been practicing yoga for more than 40 years and during most of that time, I was a very frustrated seeker looking for the magic recipe for a perfect stress-free life. I wanted to be able to do all those crazy yoga postures, live in a gorgeous body, eat pure nutritious food, sleep soundly (waking totally refreshed), be employed in an incredible, high paying intelligent job, enjoy wonderful relationships with everyone in my life including my family, and experience pure bliss every single day.

This book has been written in response to all of the above concerns and situations. I take your life seriously and wish you well in whatever path you choose up the mountains of your life. The yoga techniques offered in this book are not new and they are not mine, they belong to every human being. I humbly offer what I found in an ancient tradition that works for me; hopefully, something within these pages will work for you.

What have I learned?

- Stress is here to stay. Deal with it.
- Diets don't work unless you address your stress issues.
- Yoga postures are only the tip of the iceberg. Yoga is much deeper.
- Practicing yoga will help you manage your stress and weight issues for the rest of your life.
- Health, wealth, and happiness are created and nurtured from within.
- There are many paths up the mountain. Find what works for you. When you get to the top of the mountain: keep climbing.

Begin wherever you are.

Remember to honor your body, mind, and spirit.

Living our best life possible is all about balancing our physical, mental, emotional, and spiritual needs. Yoga is a simple, yet powerful tool available to anyone interested in seeking the truth. It is not magic. It is often difficult. Yet the joys of connecting with your true self with love and compassion will assist you in living a fuller life. Practicing yoga is an ongoing process. It is a journey of discovery and a lifetime practice.

The goal of this program is to give you the tools and ideas that I have found to help me deal with my stress and weight issues. My hope is that you will find something that will assist you in cultivating healthy habits to support your dreams, truth, and mission here on Earth.

Before we begin this journey together, I would like to know why you are reading this book?

What are you looking for? What do you need? What do you want? What is going on in your life today? (Please write your answer in the space below if this is your book, or use a separate piece of paper, or journal.)

Are you looking for a quick fix, the answer to the universe, or a painless remedy for a difficult situation?

Living a full life is not an easy task. Ask anyone who has successfully dealt with a major grief issue or trauma, an addiction, or dropped a significant amount of weight, and kept it off—it is not easy.

Diets work. Anyone can lose weight on a regimented diet, but until you get to the root of why you are not managing your stressors and weight, you will continue to be a yo-yo, spiral out of control, or have some variation of a classic eating disorder. Unless you begin to address your situation truthfully, you will continue the myth of Sisyphus, rolling your weight issues up the mountain, almost getting to the top before falling back, and then being condemned to repeat this futile event. These yoga principles offer the tools to begin to stop, look, listen, and respond to your individual situation. We are all different. One diet or system does not fit all. This program is based on the fact that you are an intelligent human being willing to acknowledge your circumstances and deal with your reality.

Now what?

Why not begin with where you are right now, in this very moment? By purchasing, or borrowing this book you have already taken the first courageous step in honestly dealing with your situation. As you explore the suggestions in this book, you may want to start thinking, meditating, and keeping a journal or notebook to deal with the following questions: What is your real mission in life? What did you really want to do as a child? What dreams do you have sitting on the back burner waiting until "the time is right"? If you were your ideal weight right now, what would you be doing? What would your life look and feel like? What is stopping you from living the life you want and need?

Also be sure to list all the stressors in your life right now, including issues in your past that are still causing stress in your life today. This includes unfinished business from cleaning out the garage, to saying *Thank you, I love you,* or *I'm sorry* to someone who needs to hear this from you (including yourself). List everything and anything that is currently stressing you. **And then take a deep long inhale, pause, and exhale.**

Let your list rest. You are about to begin changing your life by slowly incorporating ancient yoga techniques into your daily life. I urge you to take your time. There is no rush. After all these years I am still not perfect! I struggle with all my stress and weight issues every single day. This is simply a **practice**. And it takes mindful work until it becomes a healthy habit.

Do you remember learning to walk? If you watch a toddler struggle with those first few steps, fall down, get up again, fall down, get up again—their perseverance is incredible. Remember learning to read, ride a bicycle, play the piano, drive a car, sew a button on a shirt, change a diaper, or learn a new software program? The first few times were probably awkward, possibly embarrassing, and yet you kept trying. Why? You wanted a particular skill, you made a decision to learn it, and you persisted despite any negative voices inside or around you, and, over time the skill became second nature to you.

Remember that you have all the answers within. And as you begin to make positive changes in your life, one thing will lead to another, and you will have made one of the best investments in your life—your health!

Let us begin our journey to create and live our life to the best of our ability today.

Teachers open the door, but you

must enter by yourself.

~ Chinese proverb

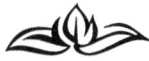

So Where's The Chocolate?

Note: *Thank you to everyone who has asked me questions when they found out that I was working on this book. I've taken the liberty of using your questions, but changing some of the details to protect your privacy.*

Questions I've Been Asked

*"Where in the world did you get this idea of **Chocolate Yoga**? Aren't people who do yoga supposed to be tall, skinny, live on air, and chant all day and night?"*

Ever since I turned fifty, people have been asking me how I keep from gaining weight. And I would say: *Just do yoga.* A few weeks later, they would come back and say: *Yoga doesn't work; you must be doing something else.* After awhile, I realized that maybe I am doing something else besides yoga postures, but what is it? That's when I started taking notes on my thought patterns, activities and eating behaviors, and realized that I am doing something different. This is not a complicated program. Anyone can do these yoga techniques. And best of all, you already have this information within you. There is nothing new in this book. You already know this yoga. All you have to do is practice it. Best of all—it's free.

"I bought this book because I thought it was a yoga diet book and you would tell me what to eat so I could get rid of this excess weight. Where are the recipes?"

The only recipes you will find are techniques for managing your stress and weight issues. If you are willing to just try some of these yoga techniques, I am sure that you will find something that resonates with you. This is simply a guide book. There is no set order.

"I don't have time to read or try anything in this book. I am too busy. Can you just give me the answer?"

Sure. Just breathe mindfully.

"You've got to be kidding. Just breathe. Your whole book is about just breathing and I won't be overweight?"

Yes. That's it. This program is based on the idea that stress and weight are flip sides of the same coin. If you manage your reaction to the stresses in your life, you will be able to manage your weight issues. And conversely, by managing your weight, you will be able to manage your stress issues. Best of all, you can do this by practicing **Chocolate Yoga**. Try it. What do you have to lose?

"What if this doesn't work?"

What is your definition of this program working for you? Until you decide to start seriously addressing your stress and weight issues, nothing will work in the long run. Yoga is all about learning to *listen*, and *managing your own life*. It's not necessarily easy. But if you don't do it, who is going to do it for you? The exercises in this book are my interpretation of yoga techniques that work for me. They may not work for you. That's OK. It's ultimately your responsibility to figure out what works for you.

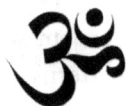

Stress and Weight
Are Flip Sides of the Same Coin

"What is the connection between stress & weight?"

I firmly believe that there is a very direct relationship between stress and weight issues. Think of stress and weight as either side of a coin. They are connected back to back. One side represents your stress issues and the other side your weight issues. There is no separation. They are attached. And that is good. Stress is here to stay, so in order to live a healthier life, we must learn to deal with our perceptions and reaction to our stress issues. The reality today is that we are witnessing worldwide obesity and starvation. The global economy has not figured out an even distribution system so that everyone has equal access in meeting their basic nutritional needs. **Chocolate Yoga** will address some of these issues on a personal, global, and spiritual level. In the meantime, it is our own personal challenge to find that delicate balance between our own personal stress and weight issues.

"What is stress?"

We use this word all the time, and yet if you ask ten people, you will most likely get ten different answers. Common definitions are: feeling overwhelmed, pressured, out-of-control, angry, strained, anxious, worried, short-tempered, pissed, annoyed, too many things to do, high blood pressure, tired, depressed, too many choices, too many demands, low-energy, manic behaviors, time crunched, and tension. The list goes on. My definition of stress is **any physiological response to any change or pressure.** Make a fist. Squeeze tightly. What happened? Did you hold your breath? Did you stop breathing? Where did you feel the tension? That is stress.

"I thought stress was a pure physical response to a situation?"

On a physical level stress triggers hormones that raise the blood sugar, which ultimately taxes the immune system. Our bodies are connected to our minds. And our minds are connected to our body. Whatever threatens our mind is perceived and registered in our body. We may choose to fight, flee or freeze, either physically, mentally or emotionally. Most of us have habitual patterns in response to the stressors in our lives. In order to anesthetize the pain of our stress, we may overeat, not eat, over-exercise, over-medicate, become a workaholic, or close ourselves off from family and friends. Over time, we will use various coping mechanisms, failing to notice how deeply they have become entrenched habits and patterns.

"I have no idea how I got this way."

It is because these changes are often so subtle, slow and seductive. We get rewarded in some way, shape or form for maintaining our defenses. We hide behind our fat, lack of fat, alcohol, drugs, money, toys, job titles, busyness, manic exercising, internet surfing, or any activity we can use to shield us from reality. Until suddenly we wake up one day totally miserable, frustrated, and fully aware that we are slowly killing ourselves.

"My doctor says my high blood pressure is due to stress and he is always giving me a new medication. Now you are telling me I just need to change my reaction?"

Yes and no. First of all, always check in with your health practitioner before making any changes to their recommendations. Secondly, do your homework. Notice when your physical symptoms appear. This may include shortness of breath, holding your breath, hyperventilating, sweating, heart palpitations, headaches, sleep disorders, diarrhea, constipation, stomach aches, susceptibility to colds, coughs or virus, muscle tensions and pain, especially in the neck, head, shoulder and lower back area. You may notice emotional responses of yelling, crying, withdrawing into silence, snapping at anyone who gets in your way, or even kicking the dog.

See if you can connect the stress issue with your weight issue. Maybe you have a friend who is always calling you for special favors which make more work for you in your already busy schedule. Every time you see their name on the caller ID you feel your blood pressure rise and your heart start beating rapidly. You brace for the request, and say, "Yes." Then you open the refrigerator and start eating non-stop. Look for connections in your behavior. See if you can open a dialog between your body and your mind. Yes, talk to yourself!

"You got to be kidding. I have stress issues all day long between family, work, friends, bills, food shopping, fixing meals, laundry, housecleaning, and everyone wants me right now. No wonder I am fat, I can't keep up with all these demands. But on the other hand I can't tell everyone to go take a long walk on a short pier. I am so stuck."

There is no easy answer or solution. I can only share with you what works for me and hopefully you will find something that works for you. We have also been taught to be helpers, and often help everyone in sight and leave nothing for ourselves.

As soon as you recognize the fine line between giving and over-giving, you will be able to honestly assess the situation, establish clear boundaries, and learn to balance all the demands in your life.

Giving, helping, and care-taking are wonderful when balanced. Food is necessary in supporting our life—when we eat too much or too little we get into trouble. The following yoga techniques will help you in creating more balance in your life, while maintaining and nourishing all your relationships, including your relationship with yourself.

"I am out of work, my teenager is giving me grief, my spouse is on my case for not working and all I can do is cry and eat. Will these yoga techniques help me get me out of this funk?"

There are no guarantees that any of these yoga techniques will work for you right now. All I can say is that sometimes when I am so down, and I wonder if my life will ever get better—I go to the library or a book store, and often find a book that gives me hope. Or I'll go do something really simple like clean under the bathroom sink. It always amazes me that when I give more motion or action to my life, I still have the same problem or situation, but I get a little bit of light and relief by physically moving. Ultimately it's your challenge to explore. Everyone and every situation are different. Not one size fits all. So I hope that something in this book resonates for you, if not, keep searching.

"I've heard you say stress is good. What do you mean?"

Well, there is *stress* and there is **STRESS**. Stress can be very motivating, challenging, and life affirming. Stress is not necessarily a *bad* or *negative* thing. It usually is not 100% positive or 100% negative.

You can use stress to grow and thrive. There is good stress, as in the pressure to get up in the morning, brush your teeth and get moving. Pressure can actually produce incredible challenges, stimulation and enthusiasm. Think of graduations, weddings, childbirth, a new job, a promotion, the holidays, traveling or a bonus check.

In the meantime start tracking your major and minor stressors and see if you can re-frame each situation. By following a **Stop, Look, Listen and Breathe** approach through the pressures in your life, you will begin to see that the way you handle stress can actually produce very real and positive changes in your life choices.

If you are always reaching for food when stressed, start by asking yourself, "What do I need to feed my body, my mind, or my spirit?" Identify what part of your body, mind or spirit is hungry. How will you **feed** that hunger? A bath? A walk? A telephone conversation? A rant and rave in your journal? A cup of tea?

Then ask, "What am I avoiding by stuffing my face and will it still be there after I finish this bag of cookies? What am I looking for? **What do I really need?**"

"But what about a major stressor, like a car accident, an unexpected family death or an international tragedy?"

There is no magic wand. I can only offer the breathing techniques in this book. Life happens. Cars crash, people die, and innocents are suddenly killed. It is important to acknowledge these major stressors in our lives and find honorable ways to express our feelings. When we feel out of control or in deep pain we may choose to repress our feelings by overeating. But that is only a momentary fix.

Pain is a signal to listen.

It is our job to figure out what to do with our pain. I personally sit, write, or walk with my grief over major stressors. Somehow I always come up with a solution to my pain. It doesn't undo the fact or reality that the car is smashed, a loved one has died, or that hundreds of people are dead. However, it gives me hope in my tears, that I can do something above and beyond drowning my sorrows by eating a whole bag of cookies.

I can contribute to my healing by reaching out and doing something—and in that action maybe the healing will touch someone else. There is no one right answer here. You have to do what resonates with you. The most important element here is to **acknowledge the pain and deal with the pain.** And yes, one could say pain, whether it is minor or major, it usually manifests as a stressor. There is no magic salve, except to breathe and listen with your heart.

"What do you mean by weight and don't we all weigh too much?"

Weight is, in reality, the measurement of pounds or kilos that we need in order to survive and hopefully thrive. Weight is only a negative if it is out of balance. Weighing too much or too little is a stress in itself. If your weight issues are holding you back physically, mentally or psychologically from creating and actualizing the life you choose to live, then you are out of balance. And someone is making a lot of money on our imbalances—the $68.7 billion diet industry. (Google 2011.) Why are we giving them our hard earned money? Just think of what we could do with $68.7 billion.

"What is homeostastis and why is it in a weight management book?"

Homeostatis is an organism's ability to maintain internal equilibrium. It may also be applied to multiple organisms, as in your entire body and the environment. Both are delicate and interconnected. Think ecology, as in a system striving for balance.

You are planning to walk with a friend at 10 AM but it's raining. Can you maintain your balance or are you going to have a melt down? Can you walk in the rain? Can you walk at the mall? Can you throw your hands up, laugh and go get coffee, or go to a movie? How we choose to deal with our stressors is always our choice.

This book is not only about weight. This is about your personal lifestyle and philosophy. These techniques may be used for the rest of your life. This is not a *lose ten pounds in seven days eating whatever you want whenever you want diet.*

"Homeostasis. Are you crazy? I am really fat? Not chubby, but really FAT. I have officially been called morbidly obese. And to make it worse, I have a crazy family and work with a bunch of nuts. And I am allergic to chocolate, how is this program going to help me?"

Good question. I don't know if this program will work for you. My first question to you is what do you want, and what do you need? I am not here to say don't be fat, or that fat isn't OK.

So I am curious. What made you pick up this book? My advice to you is to check out this program. Maybe you will find something that resonates with you. As for chocolate, keep reading. My definition of **chocolate** is pleasure. What makes you happy? What makes you sing or hum? Where is your happy place?

"My husband is skinny and I used to be really skinny. I ate anything I wanted to and never gained an ounce. Now I've hit menopause complete with a protruding belly, a muffin at my waistline, and a double chin. My legs are still OK. I am miserable. What should I do?"

Glad to hear that your legs are still OK. Listen to the language in your question. Who cares if you used to be skinny? Who cares if you hit menopause with a belly, a muffin top and a double chin. Take a deep breath and see if you can connect your body with your mind. Check out this program, but don't stop here. Keep exploring. Living life fully begins right now in this very next breath. So turn the page and see what happens.

"I don't have time to exercise. I know I should. But it becomes just one more thing on my list of things to do. Shouldn't I be getting rid of stress and not adding to it? I don't have to exercise do I?"

OK. Let's just ignore the fact that the World Health Organization estimates that 80% of all illnesses are directly or indirectly caused by stress. And let's ignore the fact that your brain thrives on physical and mental activity. Then there is—*use it or lose it.*

I once went to a cardiovascular workshop where someone in the audience asked the panelists, "What is the best exercise to do for your heart?" You could have heard a pin drop in the room. We were all waiting for the medical experts to give us the magic words. The exercise physiologist said, "The best exercise that you can do for your heart is the exercise that gives you pleasure." So I am assuming you are an adult and can think your way into the right answer for you.

"Why are you using the word management in your book? Isn't management for CEOs, people with college degrees, or full-time mothers juggling car pools, soccer, ballet, and music lessons?"

Management is for all of us. Management is the never-ending process of juggling everything in your life to achieve the best balance possible. It involves constant recalculating, total awareness, realignment, listening, practicing, working, reorganizing, changing, revising, and analyzing. Management is an ongoing full-time job, and the best manager of your life is you!

"So you're saying that if I can manage my stress issues, I can manage my weight issues?"

Yes. And by managing your weight issues you will be more present for your stress issues. This is a 24/7 management task. I am not saying that you have to be totally conscious 24/7, but you do have be breathing, listening, and paying attention for all of this to work.

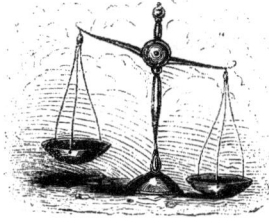

Manage Your Stress = Manage Your Weight

"You seem so even keeled, serene and peaceful. What's the deal?"

Ha! The reality check is to talk to my spouse, family, friends and coworkers. I am a real human being who gets stuck in my muck, old wounds, bad habits and knee-jerk reactions that continually pop up, embarrass and mortify me. When I remember to stop and take a few deep breaths, then I can sometimes change my behavior. And some days are better than other days. This is a reality-based practice.

"How long will this program take?"

The rest of your life. Seriously, unless you are a highly evolved master of living meditation, this is a life-time practice. I sincerely hope that you will find some pearls of wisdom within these pages or at least something that lights a spark to add some brightness and energy to your life today.

"Which came first, the stress or the weight issues?"

Does it matter? Can we blame our genes, biochemistry, the environment, the government, television, advertising or fast food? I think the two issues are so interrelated that it does not matter. Think of a teeter-totter or the astrological Libra holding the scales—with either stress issues or weight issues pulling you up or down. It just is.

"Why don't diets work?"

Oh, but they do work. Have you ever noticed that people who attempt to follow a diet—or who actually succeed in dropping weight on a prescribed set of dietary rules—crave structure? Somewhere in their lives they are out of balance and seek desperately to control something, anything. If you have ever been anorexic or bulimic, or been around someone who is, you know exactly what I am talking about. However, unless you address your real everyday stress and needs you will keep looking for another diet solution. This **Chocolate Yoga** may work or it may not. I only know it works for me.

"What about anorexia and bulimia? Are those stress-related issues?"

I have very little experience with either of these conditions. However, I do believe that as human beings we are all striving to connect with our true selves and with other people. Reactions to stressful issues take on many manifestations, consciously or unconsciously, with all sorts of behaviors—overeating, under-eating, overwork, oversleeping, sex abuse, addiction to nicotine, drugs or alcohol, shopping or overspending, gambling or gaming, internet surfing, social media or television—the list is endless. I firmly believe that if you carefully examine the endless hours spent on all of the above behaviors, they are all connected to the stressors in your life.

*"Would **Chocolate Yoga** work for people trying to put on weight?"*

I suspect if they follow the guidelines of yoga for stress and weight management they may be able to fulfill their healthy body requirements.

"Do you still read diet books and articles?"

Yes, I continue to look for magic elixirs, and I am sometimes seduced by how simple, rational, and easy any diet plan seems—until I close the book or article and return to the reality of my life. My daily stresses usually involve facing something that I really don't want to do, so on my way to do the next task, I stop in the kitchen to find some comfort, it's usually something that I just read about and it's usually on the *forbidden* or *absolutely do not eat this* list.

Oh well, I'll start that wonderful diet tomorrow morning. But tomorrow morning arrives, and guess what? Maybe I will make it to noon, but I am usually running late, or so rushed that I inevitably grab something from that forbidden/do not eat list. Oh, that's alright I tell myself, this is a very stressful week; I'll start that diet next Monday morning when all this stress is over.

Sound familiar? That's why most diets don't work in the long term. Stress and stressors are a given—whether they are big or small—as long as we are alive we will always have them. That's why a simple list of what to eat and when to eat, rarely works in the long run. Diets rarely address the stresses in our everyday life.

"Which techniques will help me with my stress issues and which ones work for my weight problem?"

I believe that stress and weight are so interconnected that I am unable to separate the two issues. A breathing exercise for stress may work equally well for a weight issue. You may take a walk to get some exercise and come home totally relaxed because you met a neighbor and had a delightful fulfilling conversation. You may also notice that you are not so hungry. So it's hard to say if the walk or the talk was more beneficial for stress or weight management.

Or let's say you were practicing your breathing exercises in the car on the way to work, and when you arrive at the office you find an unexpected crisis. Suddenly you are rolling up your sleeves and handling the situation with grace and equanimity (whereas this situation would have normally sent you running for donuts).

Were the breathing techniques you just did in the car for stress or weight management? Probably both! Think of these exercises and techniques as vitamins you take throughout the day to keep you in great shape and ready to handle any crisis or stress that rolls your way!

"Is that why you give four stress-related exercises and only one weight management suggestion at the end of each section?"

My personal experience has been that my overeating patterns are so connected to whatever is stressing me in the moment, that I cannot think clearly to choose a healthy eating response. Some of my stresses are glaringly obvious, but many are subconsciously pulling the strings of my behavior. By using these yoga techniques on my body, I can often quiet the chatter in my mind and hear the truth. If I can listen without judgment I can deal with the real issues—being tired, hungry, sad, angry, stuck, upset, hurt, vulnerable—then I can get to the root and usually figure out a healthy choice. That is why there are more stress related techniques in each section than weight management tools.

If you can continually monitor your stress levels, you will automatically be making healthier nutritional choices—and you will experience more **Chocolate Yoga** moments in your everyday life!

Chocolate Yoga is the Solution!

"What exactly is Chocolate Yoga?"

The definition of *chocolate* as we know it today is processed cocoa seeds, usually combined with sweeteners and/or flavorings.

The word *chocolate* is used in this book as a code word to mean something that fills your heart and makes you sing. **It does not need be an actual piece of chocolate.** It is what gives you pleasure. My definition of pleasure is healthy, safe, ethical and legal activities. It is that classic moment of *all is well.* It is a feeling of peace, tranquility, and joy. It is difficult to find the right words, but you know it when you feel it. That is YOUR *Chocolate Yoga.*

The classic definition of *yoga*—based on the Sanskrit word *yuj* or *yoke*—is the sense of bringing things together to join or unite. *Yoga* is a state of being *one* within your body and your mind. *Yoga* is an on-going process and a practice, it is not an end in itself.

My use of the word *yoga* is the process of mindfully using your breath to balance the body and the mind.

"I still don't get it!"

Chocolate Yoga is a feeling. It can best be described as a sense of peace and that all is well. It is that first bite of chocolate, cake or ice cream. It is that first sip of wine, cocoa or sweet iced tea. It is that sensation that just melts in your mouth and travels through your body. Of course, it usually feels so good we want more. The idea of *Chocolate Yoga* is to be able to live more in the moment so that we can totally enjoy that first bite or sip without having to eat or drink the whole thing in one big inhale.

Chocolate Yoga will help you enjoy and savor that moment so that your life is richer, fuller and more satisfying. *It is important to remember that these moments are NOT all food related.*

Chocolate Yoga can be found all around you in many ways, shapes, and forms! It may be the pleasure you get from holding an infant who is snuggling on your chest; it may be that wonderful warm feeling after a good night's sleep and the bed is warm and delicious; it may be looking at the sunlight filtering through the trees; it may be watching a dog chase a Frisbee or children playing; it may be the smell of garlic roasting from a neighboring restaurant in the evening; or taking a walk on a summer evening though the neighborhood, smelling all the barbecue grills; or the smell of flowers or a bakery. It is everywhere.

"Sounds like a lot of smelling?"

Actually, we all have dominant senses. Mine is obviously the sense of smell. Think of the other senses—hearing, seeing, touching and tasting. A *Chocolate Yoga* moment may be listening to a beautiful piece of music, singing in the car, or being at a concert. It may be seeing the sunrise or sunset. It may be massaging a loved one or using a new delicious skin cream. It might be the "wow" on that first sip of wine or that a spoonful of spaghetti sauce simmering on the stove. *Chocolate Yoga* could be all or any of the above.

Although you may not be able to hold on to that moment, the goal is to *savor* that moment and to consciously appreciate it with your whole body, mind and spirit. Think of *Chocolate Yoga* moments as *soul food*—necessary nutrients for living a richer life.

"Chocolate Yoga sounds like senses on hyperdrive. I am too busy to pay attention to every moment or everything that I am doing. Sounds like more stress and things to do."

Chocolate Yoga is anything that totally centers you in a space and place of pure happiness and bliss. By acknowledging these *moments in the moment*—you will be happier, lighter and more energetic. You will be able to make healthier choices as you ride the waves of your stressors.

"Waves of stress sounds like more Zen breathing in the moment and all is well in the universe crap."

Have you ever sat on a beach and watched the waves come in and go out? These waves continue 24/7 with or without our witnessing their action. We do not control the oceans and yet the waves continue.

This image may not work for you. Your task is to find images that resonate with you, so that you may be able to find a sense of peace, equanimity and acceptance with all that you *cannot* control.

If you get anything from this book, I hope you get the idea that you can always come back to your breath. Your breath resides in you right now and it is one of the best, instantly assessable stress and weight management tools ever created. It is figuratively and literally your best friend.

"Your yoga ideas don't seem very scientific, or even well documented."

This book is a composite of yoga techniques that I practice on and off my mat. If you need science-based evidence concerning yoga and stress management, I encourage you to go to the library, find a knowledgeable yoga teacher, or seek out reliable databases on the internet. There are on-going international efforts to prove scientifically that yoga works. If you need more technical advice, or you are interested in expanding your yoga practice, please find a teacher that resonates with you. In the meantime, enjoy your quest to seek your truth and find the techniques and paths that work for you.

"You are asking me to try these yoga techniques and see what happens? Who has time? Why should I listen to you?"

Your responsibility is to listen to yourself. I am only here to share what works for me. Your life is *your* life.

Stress is here to stay. If you adopt the attitude that stress is always changing—and take a moment to breathe between the acknowledgement of the stressor and your response—you may find yourself actually thriving on the challenge to respond appropriately.

By identifying and processing your stressors using the following yoga techniques you will be able to deal with your stress in more creative life-affirming ways and be able to successfully manage your weight.

"What do I need to remember?"

- Stress and weight are flip sides of the same coin.
- Manage your stress issues = manage your weight issues.
- *Chocolate Yoga* is the Solution (Answer).

"That's all I need?"

Actually, just breathe, smile and sing. It works and it's free!

Change is good. You go first.

~ bumper sticker

How To Use This Book

This program is designed to be flexible. It can be done individually, with a partner/friend, or in a group.

The Five Chapters

1. *Pranayama,* The Breath: Connecting the Body & the Mind

2. *Bandhas,* Energy Locks: Creating Core Heat

3. *Drishti,* The Gazing Points: Looking In & Looking Out

4. *Asanas,* The Postures: Meditation in Motion

5. *Savasana,* Rest & Relaxation: Recharging Your Batteries

Each chapter is divided in three sections:

- **Questions I've Been Asked:** A collection of actual questions about yoga from my conversations with students, friends, and people in the supermarket line.
- **Yoga Techniques for Stress and Weight Management:** Suggestions, instructions and guidance for using yoga techniques to manage your stress and weight issues.
- **Questions to Ask Yourself.**

Living Chocolate Yoga: Putting it all Together

The **Ultimate Chocolate Meditation.** This is a daily practice. It all begins and ends in chocolate!

Quick Guide for Exercises

A Guide to all the exercises above. You may copy it as a quick reference, add other ideas or use it when you travel.

Please remember that there is no set order for this practice. You may find yourself practicing the same breathing technique for weeks at a time, maybe months, it doesn't matter. The most important thing is to remain open and curious about what works for you right now—in your very next breath.

*You may want to add the following to your **Chocolate Yoga** practice:*

- a notebook or sketchbook,
- pen/pencil/markers,
- yoga/pilates/exercise mat or pad,
- comfortable clothing (including pajamas!),
- yoga belt, tie, or bathrobe sash/belt,
- clear space on an empty wall and/or a locked door for privacy,
- chair with a straight back,
- a sense of humor.

Ground Rules and Guidelines for all the exercises

Stop, Look, Listen, and Breathe. When in doubt—Breathe. Breathe. Breathe. Going deeper? Breathe. Scared? Breathe. Dizzy? Breathe. Shakey? Breathe. Remember to pause and breathe between the stimulus and your response.

Start with where you are now. Honor your body, your injuries, and your surgeries. Work with the body you have right now.

Listen to your body/mind—pain is the messenger. If you experience any sharp pains, back off, this also includes emotional pain. Take a deep breath and reassess the situation. I am assuming you are a responsible person, and if you need to, please go get professional help.

*There is no rush in **Chocolate Yoga**.* You have all the time in the world. By actually backing off and gently working with your body that you have today, you will go deeper.

Have fun, experiment, lighten up, and smile. It actually helps with the breathing!

It's okay to ask for help! Accessing health care professionals.

Sorry folks, there is no magic pill. No magic bullet, surgery, or makeover. Life is work and sometimes we need help. It's okay to ask for, and seek help. If you are a survivor of physical, sexual or emotional abuse, please seek assistance in a therapeutic setting where you can begin to create space to heal.

There are many resources and health care professionals who are trained to heal the body, mind, and spirit. Do your research and consider the following: acupuncturist, chiropractor, career coach, dance teacher, dentist, dietitian/nutritionist, gym/health club, martial arts teacher, massage therapist, meditation class, minister, nurse practitioner, personal trainer, pharmacist, physician, priest, reiki practitioner, spiritual guide, sports coach, therapist, support group, time management specialist, tai chi teacher, or yoga teacher. The bottom line: *How do you feel after being with that practitioner or leaving that coach/teacher?* Trust your gut.

There are so many wonderful ways to celebrate, balance, and nurture your body, mind, and spirit. You don't have to become anything you don't want to be. Practice listening to yourself. Practice breathing. **Seek balance and be curious** about what works and does not work for you. It's called wisdom. Remember, no one person, or system has all the answers, including you or me.

Take whatever you need or want.

Please remember that this is a *practice*. Take whatever you need or want from this book. There is nothing magic except your breath. If you continually come back to your breath, you will discover that you still have the same stress and weight issues, but that they are lighter. There is more room to breathe, move, and change the situation when you take time to really notice your truth.

The exercises that follow are simple.

We are all looking for health, wealth and happiness. Most of us are looking for that pill a day that will take the weight away and then we will be stress free! We want an instant quick fix.

But we do have an instant quick fix—it is available 24/7—it is free!

Just Breathe!

If you do not change your
direction you are likely to end up
where you are headed for.

~ Chinese proverb

... Just Breathe ...

inhale – pause – exhale– pause – inhale – pause – exhale– pause
– inhale – pause – exhale – pause – inhale – pause – exhale–
pause – inhale – pause – exhale– pause – inhale – pause –
exhale – pause – inhale – pause – exhale– pause – inhale
– pause – exhale– pause – inhale – pause – exhale – pause –
inhale – pause – exhale– pause – inhale – pause – exhale– pause
– inhale – pause – exhale – pause – inhale – pause – exhale

... Just Breathe ...

inhale – pause – exhale– pause – inhale – pause – exhale– pause
– inhale – pause – exhale – pause – inhale – pause – exhale–
pause – inhale – pause – exhale– pause – inhale – pause –
exhale – pause – inhale – pause – exhale– pause – inhale
– pause – exhale– pause – inhale – pause – exhale – pause –
inhale – pause – exhale– pause – inhale – pause – exhale– pause
– inhale – pause – exhale – pause – inhale – pause – exhale

... Just Breathe ...

Chapter 1

Pranayama

The Breath:
Connecting the Body & the Mind

Questions I've Been Asked

"Why is the breath so important?"

Breath is life. It is the first question we ask when a baby is born, *"Is it breathing?"* Then we go on to identify the sex of the baby, and count toes. At the end of life, we ask the same question, *"Is s/he still breathing?"* Breath is the foundation of life. It cannot be underestimated. It is also the foundation for practicing yoga. The body can live without food for weeks, a few days without water, but only a few minutes without air.

"What is pranayama?"

The Sanskrit word for breath is *prana* and *yama* means extension. *Pranayama* refers to yoga breathing techniques. By controlling the breath, you can begin to control and influence your mind and your body.

"There are so many different kinds of yoga breathing techniques, which one is the best?"

All of them! The word *prana* is also used to refer to the inner "life force." The deeper the quality and volume of your breath, the more vitality you will manifest. There are many breathing techniques to attain breath control.

The majority of *Pranayama* exercises involve basic combinations of: inhales; exhales; retention after the inhales; and/or retention after the exhales. Think of your breath as a musical instrument that offers many combinations of sound variations.

The most important thing in all these exercises is that you stay connected with your breath. If you feel intense constriction, deep discomfort, extreme dizziness or any pain whatsoever, back off immediately.

"I don't have time for all these fancy breathing techniques. What is the simplest most basic technique?"

My favorite technique is to simply fill the lungs on a deep inhale, hold gently for a *very* short pause, and then exhale until the lungs are completely empty. It is easy to do and the benefits are immediate. Try it right now. I guarantee you will feel better.

"How do I use my breath?"

The breath is a very powerful tool that is totally accessible to you anytime and anywhere. And it's absolutely free! It is an extremely versatile instrument. It can be used to energize, calm, and focus your body or your mind. It is your best friend—it requires no special clothes, mat or class schedule.

When you are feeling depressed, scattered, out of control, angry, scared or irritated—take a real deep breath. Try some of the breathing techniques in this book, or go exploring and find a breathing technique that works for you. Watch a baby or a young child breathing and notice how they breathe with their entire body. Use your breath wisely and mindfully to support yourself in every situation.

"Why is the breath called the mirror to the body/mind?"

Notice your breathing right now. Is it calm? Even? Smooth? Erratic? Constricted? Are you holding your breath? The breath is a reflection of the state of your body and your mind. Notice how you are breathing the next time you are upset, angry, sad or feeling pressured. Then notice your breathing the next time you are happy, peaceful, rested or laughing. The breath is an excellent barometer to measure the state of balance between your body and your mind.

"How do I monitor my breath when I am not even aware that I am breathing?"

It's a habit that you can develop over time. **Just stop wherever you are and very quietly tune into your breath.** Try this the next time you are sitting in a car, at the dinner table, in a meeting, or before you answer the phone. As you wake up in the morning, tune in to you breath. Is your breathing fast, slow, smooth, shallow, irregular, constricted or relaxed? Without passing judgment, use this information, and then take your breath to the place that you want to go.

"My mother told me to count to ten whenever I got really angry."

The technique of stopping when you are angry to take ten deep breaths has been handed down through the generations for a very good reason—**it works.** Mom was right. By pausing to mindfully breathe, the body/mind has an opportunity to check in with reality. Instead of a knee-jerk reaction to whatever is triggering the anger, you have the opportunity to stop and readjust your response.

You can even say, *"Wait, let me take a few deep breaths before I respond."* This technique can be used anytime and anywhere for any emotion or situation.

Note: *you may find yourself in an emergency situation where there is no time to stop and breathe—you need to take action with your next breath. If you are really in your body and tuned in, you will do the right thing.*

"There are many words and images for breath, which is best?"

If one looks closely at the origins of the word *breath*, it was often used interchangeably with the perception of spirit, soul, and the wind. The Greek root *pneuma* (breath) and *psychein* (to breathe), and the Latin root *spiritus* (breath) can all be linked to the words we use today—breath, life, psyche, soul, spiritual and respiratory.

I personally like the image of my *breath* as my *spirit*. One does not have to believe in the concept of a soul, to believe that the breath is a basic measurement of life force. All traditions and cultures acknowledge the importance of the breath in some manner.

Other words for breath are: *chi* (Chinese), *ha* (Hawaiian), *ki* (Japanese), *prana* (Sanskrit), *mana* (Malayo-Polynesian), *orenda* (Native American), *neshamah* (Hebrew), or *ruach* (Hebrew-Aramaic).

You may want to play with different images and see your breath as ocean waves, a river, a bubbling brook, or wind through the trees. Other images may include actually visualizing the lungs breathing, butterfly wings gently flapping or bellows gently stoking the fire within.

"I've noticed that my breath is lopsided. I usually just breathe out of my left nostril."

Most of us breathe out of a dominate side for many reasons; habit, structural (deviated septum), or allergies. As you observe your breath throughout the day, you may notice that one nostril will be more dominant than the other. Some practitioners believe alternate nostril breathing will help balance not only your breathing, but the right and left hemispheres of your brain. It is also believed that the right nostril represents the *solar* or masculine/*yang* elements, and the left nostril reflects the *lunar* or feminine/*yin* elements. There are also some systems that adhere to the idea that breathing is more dominant in one nostril than the other depending on the time of day or night. Most of us have noticed that we feel better after a good workout that forces breathing through both nostrils.

Yoga seeks balance—therefore breathing equally out of both nostrils is something to work towards, without ever forcing the breath.

"I have asthma. Just the thought of closing my mouth to breath though my nose gives me a panic attack."

Open your mouth. Breathe through your mouth. The most important part of breathing is to breathe comfortably. Only you can be the judge of your comfort level. Never push yourself to do something that doesn't feel right.

"I've heard that I am not really doing yoga unless I breathe?"

I've had many teachers tell me that **the breath is the most important element of yoga** and for many years I just ignored them. I was too busy trying to get my foot behind my head, often hyper-ventilating with frustration, or holding my breath thinking I'd get there faster. The irony is now that I've given up trying to get my foot behind my head—and I've learned to concentrate on my breathing—my foot is almost behind my head. The **breath is key to everything you do,** including practicing yoga.

"Why is breathing the most important element of yoga practice?"

It is the foundation for all of yoga. Think of your breath as the fuel that you put into your vehicle—your body. So why not create the finest fuel available to get the best mileage possible?

By using your breath wisely, you will find yourself connecting and reconnecting with your internal and external worlds. Your breath is your ticket to mindfully practicing yoga on and off the mat.

"Sometimes I sound like a wheezing turtle when I try yoga breathing, what's going on?"

It may be that you are trying too hard. Breathing should never be uncomfortable. If your breath seems strained, it is important to back off, slow down or take a break. Quite often your breath will change as you continue practicing. In the morning my breathing is usually stuffy and jerky. However, as I continue to relax and practice, my breath becomes smoother and steadier.

If you have a cold, asthma, allergies, sinus problems, very high or very low blood pressure, are pregnant or extremely overweight, on certain medications or are really upset about something—your breathing may be irregular or erratic. Check in with your health care practitioner or a seasoned yoga teacher for guidance.

"How do you do ujjayi breathing?"

Ujjayi breathing is often translated from Sanskrit as *victorious breath*. It is best demonstrated by gently blowing onto the palm of your hand as if you were fogging up a window or mirror. Now close your mouth, and do that same breath. It may sound almost like a whisper at the back of the throat. The *glottis* is slightly constricted, yet there should be no discomfort. (The glottis is the part of the larynx consisting of the vocal cords and the slit-like opening between them. It affects voice modulation through expansion or contraction.)

Some people refer to *ujjayi* breathing as wind through a tunnel, Darth Vader breath, vacuum cleaner breath, or wheezing wizards. My favorite term is ocean breath, as in the sound you hear when you put a sea shell up to your ear. Once you get into the sound and the rhythm of the breathing, it is incredibly soothing, cleansing and relaxing.

"I don't think I could do ujjayi breathing in public."

Yes, but you could do *ujjayi* breathing in the car, at home, in the bathroom, or at any moment you find yourself alone. It's okay to take deep breaths throughout the day. Just pause and do a deep inhale, holding for one second, then do a deep exhale. It feels absolutely wonderful. Once you begin, you will find yourself taking several deep breaths, relaxing your jaw, and smiling.

"What is easy breathing, as in meditation poses?"

I use *easy breathing* for instant meditation. Just find a comfortable seated position. Begin by just listening to your inhales and exhales, and then very slowly see if you can lengthen each inhale to match each exhale. I like to keep my eyes half open, but some people prefer to close their eyes.

To keep your focus on counting each breath, you can use a beaded necklace, bracelet or prayer beads. The most important and sometimes hardest element is to **stay focused on just breathing**. If you find your mind wandering, just say *inhale* as you inhale, and then say *exhale* as you exhale. Don't waste your time by beating yourself up over your mind wandering—just go back to inhaling and exhaling. Over time you will find this to be incredibly soothing and relaxing.

"Can you lose weight by just using these breathing techniques?"

Yes and no. By just becoming aware—of how fast we shovel food into our mouths without pausing to taste, chew, talk or breathe between bites—mindfully breathing may help balance your weight issues. I know that every time I consciously take a bite of food, put my eating utensil down, chew and breathe, I eat less. I am also more satiated with less food. Nourishing oneself is not just limited to the amount of calories consumed; it is connected to a much larger picture. Food is a gift and we all need to slow down and be present to receive it.

"I married into a family that eats like vacuum cleaners—they can inhale a Thanksgiving meal in less than 10 minutes. They drive me nuts. I've gained 45 pounds since I got married. What should I do?"

Put your folk down. It's the most simple and powerful awareness tool that you can use. It may be awkward at first, you may have to put your hands in your lap as you pause, take a deep breath and then pick up your fork again. Use eating as a meditation exercise.

Notice how often we mirror the people and culture around us. You may want to experiment and ask your tablemates interesting questions and see what happens. These suggestions are not an instant fix, but it will help you break the automatic pilot that so many of us are stuck in.

If it's any comfort—you are not the only one. Most of us have wolfed down our food at some point in our lives—I call it the *feed bag* and the only way I can control it is to put down my eating utensil, and take a deep inhale and exhale. Then I pick up my fork or chopsticks again and continue.

"What is the most wonderful thing about the breath?"

It is so accessible! It will give you exactly what you need when you need it. It will recharge your batteries if you are tired. It will calm you down if you are too wound up. It is the connection between your body and your mind. Think of it as this wonderful deep well or reservoir that you can draw on at any time. It is the key to tranquility, peace and living. It is available to you at any hour of the day or night. It's free and it's totally yours!

"I don't have time or energy to do any of this. What do you suggest?"

Smile. Just smile! In fact, try it right now! What happened? How do you feel? It may feel a bit silly at first, but it works! It's a simple technique that provides an instant lift and can be done anytime.

On your next inhale, feel your breath going in and on each exhale feel your face softening. Let your lips curl up slightly into a smile, as if you know the secret to the universe. The immediate benefit is that you will feel your face soften, your jaw relax, your breath flowing effortlessly. You will also feel your spirit lift and probably notice how much easier it is to greet and look people in the eye. People will begin to smile back and everyone's spirits will be lifted.

Smiling is a great stress and weight management tool!

☙✗❧

Exercises for Breathing Through Stressful Situations to Create Healthier Eating Patterns

Everyone teaches breathing exercises differently—these are just suggestions. Be open to trying different methods, knowing that the best techniques are the ones that work for you today.

These yoga breathing techniques are great for meditation—whether you have one minute or 20 minutes, they are all incredibly nurturing and energizing.

If you are pregnant, have any cardiac or lung problems (including asthma)—please consult your health care practitioner before attempting the following breathing exercises.

You may want to remove your glasses. If you are wearing contacts, please be mindful of your eye comfort.

Yoga Breathing Techniques for Stress & Weight Management

#1. Instant Stress Release 24/7

- This calming breathing technique is extremely flexible. You may choose to do a few breaths, several minutes, or go for as long as you feel comfortable. Listen to your inner voice. Let your breath be your guide.
- Choose only words or images that resonate with you.
- You may choose to keep your eyes open, closed, or just lower your eye lids halfway. Whatever you choose to do, be sure to keep your eyes soft.

Note: *If you are operating a vehicle please keep your eyes open.*

- Remember never force your breath. It's okay to stop at any time to cough, sneeze, yawn, cry, laugh and do whatever you need to stay comfortable.

Feel free to substitute or use any word or concept you choose in the following examples. This simple breathing technique works for equalizing any emotion, feeling or situation. If you are by yourself, in complete privacy, you may choose to say the words out loud.

This also works in the heat of the moment—when dealing with a car that just cut you off on the highway, or an obnoxious person. Just take a deep inhale and mentally say, *Inhale blue car that just cut me off;* pause, and then exhale and say, *Exhale blue car that just cut me off.* You will feel much better! Or you can take a deep inhale and mentally say, *Inhale Mr. X;* pause, then as you exhale say, *Exhale Mr. X.*

This also works in the middle of the night, when you wake up with that churning belly and are totally pissed off at a person, situation or incident.

You haven't changed the fact that you were cut off on the highway or that Mr. X was not very pleasant today, or that you are upset with someone—you've just equalized the tension! It does not cure the problem, but it does offer some relief, space and freedom to be open to a solution or resolution.

Of course, the deeper the angst and emotions around the situation, the more rounds of *inhale/pause/exhale* you may have to do to release your tension and find your balance in the situation.

Note: *This is not a cure all for problems, it is an adjunct therapy that also may lead you to seeking the assistance of a health care professional.*

Example A: Celebrating the Breath—*to create and increase Chocolate Yoga moments!*

> Inhale... *breath...*
> (Pause)
> Exhale... *breath...*
> (Pause)
> Inhale... *joy...*
> (Pause)
> Exhale... *joy...*
> (Pause)
> Inhale... *peace...*
> (Pause)
> Exhale... *peace...*
> (Pause)
> Inhale... *love...*
> (Pause)
> Exhale... *love...*
> (Pause)
> Inhale... *compassion...*
> (Pause)
> Exhale... *compassion...*
> (Pause)
> Inhale... *happiness...*
> (Pause)
> Exhale... *happiness...*
> (Pause)
> Inhale... *kindness...*
> (Pause)
> Exhale... *kindness...*
> (Pause)
> Inhale... *yoga...*
> (Pause)
> Exhale... *yoga...*

Note: *Your list doesn't have to be a long litany of concepts. It can just be done in a few breaths... quietly... silently as you are placed on hold on the phone; stuck in traffic; waiting in line at the store, or in the airport. This can also be an incredibly uplifting meditation as you notice all the positive elements in your life. Also note what images come to mind as you verbalize or visualize each concept.*

Example B: Seeking Balance and Equilibrium—*to create more space for Chocolate Yoga.*

Note: *A specific name works best in all of the following examples! You may make these words as personal as you choose, by actually naming your spouse, child, friend or anyone that comes to mind. This meditation is very healing for any situation.*

> Inhale... *spouse...*
> (Pause)
> Exhale... *spouse...*
> (Pause)
> Inhale... *taxes...*
> (Pause)
> Exhale... *taxes...*
> (Pause)
> Inhale... *my boss...*
> (Pause)
> Exhale... *my boss...*
> (Pause)
> Inhale... *rude person on the phone...*
> (Pause)
> Exhale... *rude person on the phone...*
> (Pause)
> Inhale... *family...*
> (Pause)
> Exhale... *family...*
> (Pause)
> Inhale... *my things to do list...*
> (Pause)
> Exhale... *my things to do list...*
> (Pause)
> Inhale... *friends...*
> (Pause)
> Exhale... *friends...*
> (Pause)
> Inhale... *loving kindness...*
> (Pause)
> Exhale... *loving kindness...*
> (Pause)
> Inhale... *peace...*
> (Pause)
> Exhale... *peace...*

Note: *Sometimes I call this breathing exercise the **band-aid** because it soothes my ruffled feathers and offers some comfort when I am hurt, tired, angry or any other emotion that is getting in the way of creating a **Chocolate Yoga** moment.*

Example C: Looking out the Window—*also a great one to do while driving a car! It will help you keep focused and on task.*

> Inhale... *flowers...*
> (Pause)
> Exhale... *flowers...*
> (Pause)
> Inhale... *pine trees...*
> (Pause)
> Exhale... *pine trees...*
> (Pause)
> Inhale... *squirrel in the tree...*
> (Pause)
> Exhale... *squirrel in the tree...*
> (Pause)
> Inhale... *clouds...*
> (Pause)
> Exhale... *clouds...*
> (Pause)
> Inhale... *truck passing by...*
> (Pause)
> Exhale... *truck passing by...*
> (Pause)
> Inhale... *airplane overhead...*
> (Pause)
> Exhale... *airplane overhead...*
> (Pause)
> Inhale... *sunshine...*
> (Pause)
> Exhale... *sunshine...*

Note: *This is also a great exercise to do when you are stuck waiting at a doctor's office, an airport or in any line. It gives me a sense of connection to all the seemingly disconnected elements of the moment. I also start to notice things that I didn't see before. It is incredibly soothing and helps me stay focused in the moment.*

Example D: I am… *Affirmations are very personal and powerful when based on one's true values.*

Note: *The following example is just a suggestion. Many people feel that affirmations are a waste of time and give false hope. I find them to be great therapy when I am feeling blue, all alone, and there are no cookies within reach.*

> Inhale… *I am peaceful…*
> (Pause)
> Exhale… *I am peaceful…*
> (Pause)
> Inhale… *I am beautiful…*
> (Pause)
> Exhale… *I am beautiful…*
> (Pause)
> Inhale… *I am compassionate…*
> (Pause)
> Exhale… *I am compassionate…*
> (Pause)
> Inhale… *I am energetic…*
> (Pause)
> Exhale… *I am energetic…*
> (Pause)
> Inhale… *I am creative…*
> (Pause)
> Exhale… *I am creative…*
> (Pause)
> Inhale… *I am happy…*
> (Pause)
> Exhale… *I am happy…*

Note: *Remember to have fun with this too. It's OK to laugh. I once tried this breathing visualization with "I am starving… I am so hungry… I am going to faint from hunger." I wound up laughing and ended up doing a chore that needed to be done!*

#2. *Nadi Shodhana*—Alternate Nostril Breathing

Nadi Shodhana is often translated from Sanskrit as *sweet breath*. *Nadi* refers to the channels that the *prana* (breath, life force, energy) use to travel up and down the spine, and *Shodhana* means *cleansing*. This practice is very soothing and often brings a sense of balance and equilibrium to the body, and hence will calm the mind.

1. Find a comfortable position that will keep your spine erect.

2. Place your right index and middle finger on the bridge of your nose between your eyebrows. Gently place your thumb on your right nostril.

   Some people find it more comfortable to place the middle finger on the bridge of the nose and use two fingers on each side to close the nostril. Try it both ways or make up something that works for you.

3. Close the left nostril with your ring finger and inhale through the right nostril for the count of five.

4. Pause for one second, and then release the left nostril as you close the right nostril with your thumb. Completely exhale through your left nostril.

5. Alternate sides, slowly working up to five sets on each side. Never force the breath. You will find your capacity will increase over time.

Note: *Sometimes this breathing exercise is difficult to do if you have a sinus infection, cold or asthma, so please be very gentle.*

༄

#3. *Ujjayi Breathing*—Victorious Breath

Ujjayi breathing creates a deep resonant sound at the back of the throat, as you close the mouth and breathe through the nose. If for any reason this breathing becomes uncomfortable, please remember to open your mouth. ***Chocolate Yoga*** is about releasing stress, not creating more stress.

1. The best way to understand this technique is to bring your hand about three inches in front of your mouth, gently blow onto the palm of your hand, making the sound *ha* as if you were fogging up a cold window.

2. Now close your mouth. Inhale, then exhale gently making that same *ha* sound completely through your nose.

   You will feel the glottis in the back of the throat constrict as the breath moves up the throat.

3. By keeping a soft smile on your lips, you will find your jaw relaxing and the breath moving slowly and smoothly.

The slight constriction in the back of the throat produces a sound that has often been compared to listening to gentle waves along the shoreline, or the wind blowing through the trees. On a humorous note it aslo has been called Darth Vader breath, vacuum cleaner breath, or wheezing wizards.

Ujjayi breathing can be done anytime and anywhere. It is incredibly soothing if you are feeling rattled, stressed or fatigued. You can also practice this breathing when you are doing any activity from walking or golfing to chopping vegetables! Listening to your inhales and exhales may also turn your *breathing exercise* into an instant meditation! Even a few cleansing breaths will bring immediate results.

❧⤬❧

#4. *Kalapathi, Kapala-bhati* or *Kapalabhati*—Skull-Shining-Breathing

Sometimes referred to as controlled hyper-ventilation.

This is a great exercise to get your engine started and energize your body. It can also lead to light-headiness or dizziness, which may or may not be appealing. Keep your eyes softly focused as you do this exercise.

1. Sit in a comfortable position with your spine as straight as possible.
2. Relax the abdomen, take a deep inhale, then exhale.
3. Then inhale sharply and quickly pull the belly button towards your spine. The mouth remains gently closed as the abdominal muscles raise the diaphragm and push the air out of the lungs.

Begin with three to ten rapid inhalations, then exhale slowly and breathe normally. Remember to keep your mouth gently closed and your face relaxed.

Gradually work up to a count of sixty. Remember there is no rush. Listen carefully to your body and it will guide you.

⤬

#5. Yoga Breathing Technique for Weight Management

Put Your Fork (or Drink) Down and Take a Deep Breath

This is the ultimate weight management tool and is very challenging for me to follow—but it works! I find myself calmer, fuller and satiated with less food. After eating a small bite of food or sipping a beverage, put your eating utensil or drink DOWN, and take a COMPLETE inhale, pause, and exhale.

This is so astoundingly simple you will probably find yourself laughing and saying, "Well, duh!" One of my friends folded a 3x5 card and placed it on the dining room table in front of her dinner plate. As a reminder to slow down, she wrote in bold letters: **INHALE, PAUSE, EXHALE, PAUSE, INHALE, PAUSE, EXHALE, PAUSE, INHALE, PAUSE, EXHALE.** It works.

Please don't underestimate the power of this very simple technique. If I am eating alone, I will sometimes get up after 15 minutes and put a load of laundry in the washing machine, then get side tracked into doing something else. After five minutes I wander back to the table and I am usually surprised that I am no longer hungry! The good news is that I wrap up my dinner leftovers and lunch is ready for the next day!

Notice what happens during banquets or long dinner parties, when there is space and time between courses. When you are eating slowly, talking, listening and taking sips of a drink in a social situation, you may notice that you are feeling physically, emotionally and socially fulfilled. If it is a stressful situation you may want to eat and drink less, simply to avoid further problems. When you get home be sure to eat and drink something that is soothing and nurturing.

Or if you suddenly find yourself wanting to eat the entire refrigerator, freezer, and/or pantry, you may want to pause and do a breathing exercise, put your feet up the wall, write in your journal, take a walk, or do *kalapathi* until you start laughing. Then take a deep breath and move on.

Although a lot of diet literature recommends that we eat something before going to a social function. I don't. However, I would snack before going if I were pregnant, diabetic or absolutely knew that there would be nothing to eat. I like to get real clear on why I am going. If it's a social occasion then the food is a perk. I've always found something good to eat and if I am going to a social event just to eat—then I am going for the wrong reason. I am one of those people who love buffets. I always get full but never stuffed. I love to walk around, look at everything and then taste the highlights. I don't taste everything. And if the buffet looks like too much, or too over the hill—I order *a la carte.* It works for me.

The bottom line comes down to tuning in to your breathing. By using your breath as a guide, you will be able to make healthier and happier nutritional choices. By pausing between breaths, you have a moment to listen to the voices in your head, and really hear what is going on.

For some of us, it sometimes takes a few minutes to unravel the discussion between, "Should I order the salad or the chili?" And there is always the voice that says, "Give me a break! People are starving all over the world and I'm having a major peace talk between the salad and the chili?" Take some deep breaths and you will be able to make the best decision for you. Maybe you can order half portions of both? Or split the meal with a friend? Or take the leftovers home for tomorrow. Or just have a salad. Or just have the chili.

Please, remember that everything is always changing. And that is what breathing is all about. **Take a deep breath and move on.**

Questions to Ask Yourself

Am I aware of breathing right now?

What would happen if the next time I get into a difficult situation, I would just stop and take three deep inhales and exhales?

Why wait for a difficult situation? Take three deep inhales and exhales, right now. What happened?

What can I let go of right now?

When the breath wanders, the mind is unsteady. But when the breath is calmed, the mind too will be still, and the yogi achieves long life. Therefore, one should learn to control the breath.

~ Svatmarama, Hatha Yoga Pradipika

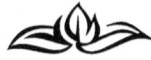

This is the Foundation!

Inhale

Pause

Exhale

Pause

Inhale

Pause

Exhale

Pause

Inhale

Pause

Exhale

Pause

Inhale

Pause

Exhale

... Creating Core Energy ...

energy locks creating core heat gates vortexes internal lifts
isometric contractions centering energy locks creating core
heat gates vortexes internal lifts isometric contractions
centering energy locks creating core heat gates vortexes
internal lifts isometric contractions centering energy locks
creating core heat gates vortexes internal lifts isometric
contractions centering energy locks creating core heat gates
vortexes internal lifts isometric contractions centering

... Centering ...

energy locks creating core heat gates vortexes internal lifts
isometric contractions centering energy locks creating core
heat gates vortexes internal lifts isometric contractions
centering energy locks creating core heat gates vortexes
internal lifts isometric contractions centering energy locks
creating core heat gates vortexes internal lifts isometric
contractions centering energy locks creating core heat gates
vortexes internal lifts isometric contractions centering

... Just Breathe ...

Chapter 2

Bandhas

Energy Locks:
Creating Core Heat

Questions I've Been Asked

"What is a bandha?"

A *bandha* in simple western terms is an internal *isometric contraction*. Bandhas are often referred to as *internal lifts, locks, energy centers, valves, gates, power centers, energetic vortexes,* or *power holds.* These energetic centers work in tandem with the breath to create the reality of truly being—physically, mentally, emotionally and spiritually centered.

The three *bandhas* discussed here can be practiced separately, or integrated together. They offer additional support for the physical body as they assist in moving energy up and down the spine. The irony of practicing these *bandhas*, are that one does not squeeze and hold tight, but that one applies just enough pressure and tension to actually engage the contraction. The *bandhas* are often subtle and elusive, yet with practice, they will lift your body, mind, and spirit.

"What is mulabandha?"

Mulabandha is often referred to as the *root lock.* In females, it is the perineum muscle lifted at the top of the cervix. It is often comparable to doing pelvic floor exercises, or *Kegels. Mulabandha* involves lifting the perineal muscle (the area between the genitals and the anus). It is simply that contraction one feels when you need to urinate and there is no bathroom in sight.

You may practice this *bandha* the next time you go to the bathroom. Simply stop urinating midstream, without contracting the buttocks or holding your breath. You can also practice it when doing yoga postures, standing in line, or seated in a car. Simply inhale, and then slowly exhale as you pull up and lift the pelvic floor.

This may seem anatomically challenging at first, but the more you practice, you will begin to feel a growing sense of lightness in your physical body. It is important to keep breathing, and stay focused as you move through any of these techniques. By identifying and isolating the correct muscles you can build strength, tone and control from within.

"How is this mulabandha going to help with stress and weight?"

This powerful tool with bring a sense of balance and strength from within your body and hence to your mind. I find this yoga technique incredibly useful for centering me and getting my mind back into my body. When I find myself distracted, unbalanced or *off-center*, by simply lifting *mulabandha*, the root lock instantly makes me take a deep breath and recalibrate. Think of it as an internal GPS (global positioning system) or a Zen clunk on the head! With a little practice you will be surprised at how much easier it is to pause, and make a healthier choice concerning responding to the stress or weight issue you are currently dealing with.

"What is uddiyana bandha?"

My favorite Sanskrit translation of *uddiyana bandha* is *flying upward*. The belly button moves toward the spinal column as the diaphragm lifts. This internal lift is done on the exhale, keeping the belly softly tucked in and still, rather than extended and protruded outward. It is a very subtle contraction, not a hard suck in the belly action.

The abdominal contraction squeezes the muscles and actually lifts the diagram and at the same time subtly engages *mulabandha* (the root lock). There is often a sensation of generating heat within, as your breath circulates around the belly and abdomen, you will begin to feel energy radiating from the inside.

Uddiyana bandha can be practiced anytime and anywhere. It will begin to tone the abdominal muscles, which in turn will strengthen the lower back muscles. It is a wonderful technique for feeling grounded, centered and energetic. Sometimes it is referred to as *fire in the belly*, *hara* (Japanese), *dan tien* (Chinese), core strength or gut strength as in *s/he has guts*. Think of it as your passion and energy center that will assist you in moving toward your goals.

"What is jalandhara bandha?"

Jalandhara Bandha is often described as a *chin lock*. The chin drops forward as it gently presses into the collarbone. This gives the neck an incredible stretch, and when coupled with breathing mindfully, often provides instant tension relief. This is also a great *bandha* to do when you've been sitting for hours, especially staring non-stop at a computer monitor, television, or movie screen.

Just take a nice deep inhale, and slowly exhale as your chin gently drops toward your collar bone. Continue breathing as you let your inhales and your exhales soften your face, especially the eyes and the jaw muscles. When you are ready to release the neck, simply inhale as you lift the chin slowly back to its normal position.

You will notice that *Jalandhara bandha* also happens naturally in many yoga postures—including shoulder-stand, forward fold, and many of the seated meditation poses. As you practice these *bandhas* you will find many opportunities to weave them in and out of your daily life and routines.

"What is maha bandha?"

Maha bandha is when *mulabandha, uddiyana bandha,* and *jalandhara bandha* are all held simultaneously. It is also called *The Great Lock,* and is a calming, yet powerful posture. This *bandha* is usually easiest when practiced in a seated position, although there are a few yoga postures that could support engaging all three *bandhas* at once. This is one of the best postures I know to practice when squished into a car or an airplane seat (unless you are the driver or pilot).

"Are the bandhas physical or energetic?"

Practicing the *bandhas* begins on the physical level because you have to start at *base camp,* which is the physical body. By engaging and coordinating the *bandhas* with your breath, the deeper you will travel into the energetic bodies. These energy bodies are called *koshas* and are often referred to as layers or sheaths of awareness. All of this takes practice and time. Remember, this is a lifetime practice and like the weather, it will change over time.

"These bandha things sound really strange, almost weird and unnatural, what's the deal?"

The awkwardness often comes from trying to find the right words to describe an internal experience. We sometimes get in the way of trying to explain everything, making things more complicated than they really need to be. The most important thing to remember is to never push or put additional strain on the body while engaging these locks.

As you work with yoga breathing, postures, gazing points and internal contractions you will begin to feel what the ancient yogis have lived and taught for years. It is all about moving energy in and out.

Just take baby steps. This is not an instant overnight practice. Enjoy the exploration. Ride the waves. Just remember it is like love, you know it when you feel it.

"While practicing the chin lock (jalandhara bandha), sitting with my back against the wall trying to meditate, I suddenly felt as if I

couldn't breathe. My throat felt choked and my double chin got in the way. What's going on?"

Rule number one, if you can't breathe comfortably, back off! Listen to your body, honor your body, and most of all keep breathing. For whatever reason, you went too far and the best thing to do is to release the posture as slowly, smoothly and gracefully as possible.

Many of us hold tension in the neck and shoulder areas, so it is very important to breathe gently into these areas allowing them to soften.

Practicing yoga is about learning to listen to the truth, and following that path. This includes the physical body.

The flexibility in practicing yoga is to try different things and evaluate them in the moment. Being able to change course as new information is being received in the moment is being truly flexible! Remember to always ease in and out of every posture as mindfully as possible.

"Can I practice these isometric contractions during the day?"

You can incorporate all of the above into the activities of your daily life. I try to practice these *bandhas* whenever I think of them throughout the day—whether it is walking the dog, standing in line, washing dishes, or before I go to sleep.

Mulabandha is basically a *Kegel* for women and a perineal lift for men. You can practice this *bandha* every time you go to the bathroom. One woman I know spends much of her day in the car and says that she gets an instant physical and psychological lift by challenging herself to practice several times an hour, using highway mileage markers as visual cues to practice.

Uddiyana bandha is a great practice to do while sitting in a chair for long periods of time, just pull your belly button toward your spine. It has also been described as tucking in the tummy as you try to zip up a pair of really tight jeans. Smile and keep breathing!

The chin lock, *Jalandhara bandha,* is a bit more challenging to practice during the day and definitely **NOT while you are driving!** However, if you are the passenger or waiting at a long stoplight, there is nothing to stop you from sitting up real straight and tall, tucking your chin gently into your collarbone, and breathing.

Sometimes my neck screams for a stretch—almost like a yawn—I just have to do it. The more you practice these locks, the more you'll find yourself doing them throughout the day.

"Can I get hurt doing these bandhas?"

If you proceed slowly and carefully, continually listening to your body, you will be fine. Some people may experience an energy surge that may be welcomed with great joy or great fear. Sometimes the truth is scary and change can be uncomfortable. If this happens to you, challenge yourself to honestly address that fear within you. You may also want to seek the wisdom of other yoga books, an experienced yoga teacher, or a health practitioner.

"I am in perimenopause. The last thing I need to do is create more core heat, I have enough heat to light up a small city!"

While in perimenopause, my experience with practicing the *bandhas* was that they actually helped me with urinary incontinence, belly fat, and stabilizing my double chin. It may be helpful to experiment with the *bandhas* during cooler periods and not in the middle of a hot flash. I would seek the knowledge of a health practitioner and always come back to your own inner wisdom.

There is no guarantee that says any of these practices will give you instant relief from anything that ails you, they are just ideas that may create more balance in your life. If something doesn't work or feel right, please toss it with the understanding that it may work for you at a later date. It is wise to keep the doors open to old and new ideas.

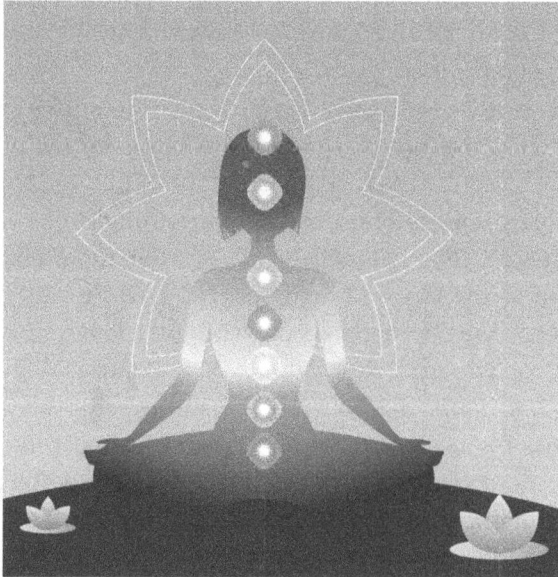

"How are these bandhas related to the chakras?"

There are seven invisible energy wheels called *chakras* that start at the base of the spine and move up the body through the top of the head. A good way to visualize these wheels is to see them as seven separate disks spinning horizontally from the center of the body.

Mulabandha is closely related to the root *chakra, muladhar. Uddiyana bandha* is connected to the *chakra* located in the solar plexus area near the *Manipur chakra. Jalandhara bandha* at the base of the throat, is located at the *Vishuddha chakra.*

These *chakras* are often referred to as *vortexes.* They are responsible for moving *prana* (life force) up and down throughout the body creating and maintaining internal balance, health, and equilibrium. Think of the breath moving up and down and all around the body, checking everything, making sure that each part is well oiled, fed, rested, happy, safe and warm.

Imagine the *chakras* spinning their colors like water wheels pouring the breath down into the next pool to keep the water moving smoothly. When there is a breakdown in one of the wheels or the pump house, the whole system is affected. Hence one of the goals of practicing yoga is to bring all the internal and external bodies into balance and harmony.

Note: *Different yoga traditions may vary in describing the exact number and location of the individual chakras.*

"What is the best bandha to concentrate on, where should I start?"

You may want to read through the following exercises and just pick one to try for a week. See what happens. All of these exercises are just suggestions for increasing our mindfulness and creating more opportunity to experience **Chocolate Yoga!**

Increasing Core Energy for Stress & Weight Management

1. *Mulabandha* (Root Lock)
2. *Uddiyana Bandha* (Flying Upward)
3. *Jalandhara Bandha* (The Chin Lock)
4. *Mahabandha* (The Great Lock) and Creating Grace Within
5. *Walking Tall* as the Ultimate Weight Management System

#1. *Mulabandha* (Root Lock)

WHO: Anyone can do this.

WHAT: *Mulabandha* is described graphically as *stop urinating mid-stream,* and *contract the perineum without squeezing the buttocks.*

WHERE: The joy of *mulabandha* is that it can be practiced anywhere. It offers internal support for any posture you are doing—whether you are in a yoga pose, standing in line, sitting in a car or walking the dog.

WHEN: *Mulabandha* can be done at any time. It is a good healthy habit to practice throughout the day, whenever you think of it. One can create this good habit by practicing it every time you go to the bathroom. This toilet meditation makes it a great mini-meditation focus for all of us who are *too busy to meditate.*

WHY: This posture builds inner physical, mental and emotional strength. I practice this every time I urinate and I am personally convinced it has helped me maintain a healthy pelvic floor.

HOW: Simply inhale and pause. As you exhale, simultaneously pull, lift and gently squeeze the pelvic floor upward toward the inner core of your body. Or just pretend that you have to urinate and then squeeze and lift. You will probably feel a surge of warm energy in the pelvic area, almost as if a current of electrical energy is being generated. Be sure not to hold your breath—let your inhales deepen and lengthen as you gently squeeze and lift the perineum. While practicing any of the *bandhas,* be sure to release slowly and mindfully.

᠁ᢍᢍᢍ

#2. *Uddiyana Bandha* (Flying Upward)

WHO: Most people can do this posture—unless you are pregnant or have recently had abdominal surgery (or this simply does not feel right). If you have any concerns, please seek professional medical advice before proceeding. Take your time and work with the body you have today.

WHAT: *Uddiyana bandha* is often referred to as *engaging the external obliques*, or *tucking in your gut to zip up a tight pair of jeans*. By internally lifting the belly button and pulling it toward the spine, the abdomen pulls in and upward; hence the Sanskrit translation and image of *flying upward.*

WHERE: *Uddiyana bandha* is a very subtle, yet powerful core lift that can be done anywhere, on or off your yoga mat. Simply stand up straight, inhale, pause, and on the exhale, pull the belly button toward the spine. You will feel the spine elongating as you stand up even straighter. Be sure to keep the shoulders down and pulled away from your ears. This is also a wonderful *bandha* to practice when you are sitting in a chair, especially at a computer, in the car or at the dinner table. It brings instant focus and attention to your core, which will make you feel more centered and grounded.

This is also an excellent exercise to practice as you are walking. Notice the difference when you are just walking along. Then engage *Uddhiyana bandha* by tucking the belly in and rolling the shoulders down and away from the ears. You will feel your spine lengthen and will find yourself walking taller, more centered and balanced.

WHEN: *Uddiyana bandha* can be practiced anytime, but preferably not on a full stomach. This is a lifetime practice and the simple action of *pulling the belly button to the spine* is usually safe and can be practiced comfortably throughout the day.

There are several intense variations of this *bandha* that are usually done in the morning before eating. They involve a more vigorous rolling of the abdominal muscles around in the pelvic cavity, in conjunction with certain breathing techniques. It is best to learn these skills under the guidance of a skilled practitioner or teacher. There are also excellent resources available online and in many yoga books.

WHY: This is a very subtle contraction that will begin to tone and strengthen the abdominal muscles and the lower back muscles. Eventually *mulabandha,* the root lock, will work in tandem and strengthen the entire abdominal core area. This *bandha* also lifts the diaphragm and will contribute to deeper, smoother and more rhythmic breathing.

HOW: Inhale, pause, and then on the exhale, lift and pull the belly button toward the spine. One way to tune into this motion is to lie down with your back on the floor or on a firm bed. Place your right or left hand gently over your belly button. Inhale. Pause. Exhale and let your hand feel the belly as it contracts and pulls toward the spine. It is very similar to doing a *pelvic tilt,* which is excellent for strengthening the front and the back muscles. It always amazes me how one little change—tucking in the belly—can bring a sense of equilibrium, centeredness and poise to one's body.

ᴑᴥᴥᴑ

#3. *Jalandhara Bandha* (The Chin Lock)

WHO: Anyone can do this posture—unless you have had recent shoulder, neck, thyroid, or eye surgery. If you have any questions or hesitations, please consult a medical professional for advice before proceeding.

WHAT: *Jalandhara bandha* is often referred to as the *chin lock.*

WHERE: Absolutely **DO NOT** do this *bandha* while driving a vehicle, operating heavy equipment, or at any other time where you need to keep your head upright for safety reasons.

As with all yoga postures and positions it is always your responsibility to tune into your body—while being aware of your surroundings. All of these yoga techniques will cultivate increased awareness and mindfulness in your everyday life. As you practice, you will notice that you are automatically paying more attention to your inner and outer worlds, and with that awareness you will create more opportunities for living **Chocolate Yoga.**

WHEN: This *bandha* happens spontaneously and naturally with many yoga postures including the shoulder stand, forward fold, and some seated meditation poses. It can also be done as you lie on the floor with your legs up the wall. (See the *Asana* [posture] section.)

This *bandha* may be done by itself or in conjunction with *Mulabandha* and/or *Uddiyana Bandha.*

WHY: There are several theories as to why this *bandha* is so important. One is that it stimulates the para-thyroid and helps to regulate metabolism. Another theory is that it gently constricts the throat *chakra,* hence forcing the *prana* (breath) to circulate around and spiral up and down the spine. Another theory is that this *bandha* strengthens the back of the neck and stretches out the top seven vertebrae in the neck area, which tends to compress as we age. The main reason I love this *bandha* is that it feels so good.

HOW: Simply sit up as straight as you can and take a deep inhale. Exhale as you gently drop the chin towards the collarbone. Continue inhaling and exhaling—feel your face soften, especially the area around the eyes, ears and jaw muscles. Send your breath to the back of the neck and down the shoulders, be sure to pull your shoulders gently away from your ears.

Quite often when you relax the neck, you will discover that other parts of your body respond positively. Use your inhales to be aware of any areas of constriction or tightness. Let your exhales soothe, smooth and relax any areas of tension. Feel any internal sharp edges becoming round and smooth as your breath circulates throughout your body. When you are ready to release the neck, simply inhale as you lift the chin slowly back to its normal position. Feel yourself sitting up straighter or standing up taller. You may even be smiling!

#4. *Maha Bandha* (The Great Lock) Creating Grace Within

This posture is very powerful and gratifying to practice. I like to sit cross-legged on the floor with my back against the wall. The wall offers firm support and at the same time keeps my spine elongated; which in turn, helps me breathe up and down my spine and into my back. If I am having a rough day or having a hard time focusing, I'll play soft classical music which seems to help me settle into the posture and stay longer than I had planned.

This is also a powerful posture to do as you are saying grace before eating—just sitting quietly with your head bowed toward your chin.

This posture will release tension in the neck and shoulder area and create a sense of stillness and peace as you center your body and mind before eating. I often refer to this posture as *the pause that refreshes*, because I can feel tranquility within seconds—in a busy restaurant, at a dinner party or sitting at the kitchen table after a busy day.

- Sit upright in a comfortable position with your spine as straight as possible.
- Begin inhaling and exhaling slowly.
- See if you can elongate the inhales, so that they match the exhales in length of time.
- Relax the facial muscles, especially the jaw and tongue, and keep the eyes softly focused on a *drishti* gazing point. (Tip of the nose, fingers or hands.)
- As you begin the next inhale, gently squeeze the perineal muscle (*Mulabandha*), followed by lifting the belly button and gently pulling it toward the spine (*Uddhiyana Bandha*), as the chin drops towards the collarbone (*Jalandhara Bandha*). This is *The Great Lock* where all three *bandhas* are actively engaged.
- Continue deepening your inhales, pauses, and exhales.
- Feel your breath moving up and down your spine.
- Pull the shoulders down away from the ears, as you open and expand the chest and lungs.
- Enjoy the sensation of warmth, heat, calm and lightness.
- Stay here for as long as you are comfortable.
- When you are ready to release the posture, be sure to take your time. On an inhale, release the chin and let it rise slowly back into its everyday position. As you exhale, let the belly soften and relax. Then very slowly release the perineal muscle, and take a few deep inhales and exhales.
- Slowly shake out your legs. Do a few neck rolls. Drop your right ear to your right shoulder and then your left ear to your left shoulder to release any tension left in the upper body. Then with a soft sweet smile, take that gift of peace and tranquility with you as you move on into your next activity.

#5. Walking Tall as the Ultimate Weight Management System

How can something so simple be so powerful? The next time you get up out of your chair and walk, notice how you are moving. Now stop.

- Stand up as tall and straight as you can.
- Roll your shoulders down and away from your ears, let your arms lengthen at your sides, feel your finger tips moving towards the floor as your chest and heart open.
- Slowly tuck your pelvis in—belly button toward the spine and drop your sit bones.
- Squeeze your thighs and feel your knee caps lift up.
- Lift the toes up towards your face and then slowly release them to the floor.
- Starting with your feet firmly planted on the ground, move your attention mindfully up the body, squeezing the thighs, and pulling the belly button towards the spine.
- Feel the chest lift as your shoulders roll away from your ears.

Yes, do it again. Roll your shoulders back from your ears. Do not under-estimate this simple gesture. You will be amazed at how quickly we revert back into hunching forward over the car steering wheel, the computer work station, or a meal.

The more you do this simple shoulder roll, the easier you will find your breath moving up and down your spine.

Pretend I am standing behind you, gently pulling your hair at the top of your head to give you one more inch of height! Feel your face softening as you start to smile. Now gently holding that beautiful tallness, begin walking. Feel your breath slowly moving you forward with perfect poise, purpose and alignment.

So where is the weight management?

When you are moving with intention, radiating peace, love and tranquility—you will find it impossible to stuff your face with any type of food or drink that is not going to support this serenity. You will also find a sense of equanimity as your feet are grounded on the earth and the crown of your head is moving toward the sky.

This posture starts with the physical, clears the mind, and connects to you to your inner being. It is very spiritual. And if you think this is too *airy-fairy,* try it in a tense situation. See if this technique works as you approach a long line that you must stand in, or you need to confront a difficult person, or situation.

When you relax the entire body into stillness with awareness, you will be able to make wiser decisions and choices. The most wonderful outcome of this practice is that it works wonders and everyone benefits, especially you!

Getting very practical: This Walking Tall technique always works for me when I am facing a buffet line, or am at a party or restaurant with many choices layered on top of social pressure, noise and other distractions.

Many of us lose our bodies as we walk into a supermarket or gaze at a menu at a restaurant. We are so out of touch with our core being, that we can be swayed by advertisements, glitzy displays and what someone else is ordering.

By using this technique, you will find yourself continually circling back to your core being. With practice, you will be able to carry on a conversation and at the same time listen to what you really want and need. This takes practice, but instead of dreading a situation, you can use all these opportunities to sharpen your skill levels and use it every day to create more **Chocolate Yoga** moments in your life!

Questions to Ask Yourself

What would happen if I just sat up straight and tall right now, and tilted my head down so that my chin was resting on my collar bone?

Can I soften my eyes and roll my shoulders away from my ears?

Can I gently pull my belly button towards my spine and actually hear myself breathing?

What can I let go of right now?

99% practice, 1% theory.

~ Sri K. Pattabhi Jois

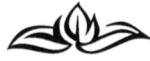

This is the Foundation!

Inhale

Pause

Exhale

Pause

Inhale

Pause

Exhale

Pause

Inhale

Pause

Exhale

Pause

Inhale

Pause

Exhale

... Gazing Points ...

gazing points looking in looking out see the truth hear the truth smell the truth touch the truth feel and sense the truth internal external balance gazing points looking in looking out see the truth hear the truth smell the truth touch the truth feel and sense the truth internal external balance gazing points looking in looking out see the truth hear the truth smell the truth touch the truth feel and sense the truth internal external balance gazing points looking in looking out see the truth

... See The Truth ...

gazing points looking in looking out see the truth hear the truth smell the truth touch the truth feel and sense the truth internal external balance gazing points looking in looking out see the truth hear the truth smell the truth touch the truth feel and sense the truth internal external balance gazing points looking in looking out see the truth hear the truth smell the truth touch the truth feel and sense the truth internal external balance gazing points looking in looking out see the truth

... Just Breathe ...

Chapter 3

Drishti

The Gazing Points:
Looking In & Looking Out

Questions I've Been Asked

"What is drishti?"

The *drishti* refers to your gaze. It has also been translated and interpreted to mean *viewpoint* or *opinion*. As in any practice and philosophy there are many layers of interpretation. On a very physical level, *drishti* literally refers to where your eyes are looking.

The eyes can be used to assist with achieving internal and external balance. This is a powerful tool that you can use to focus on where you are at this very moment, and where you want to go. Example: *I really want to do this leg lift, so if I move my eyes in the direction I want my leg to go, my leg will follow.*

It can also be used as an intention and an extension point. Example: *I can see I have three things that need immediate attention, but the most pressing task is really the second one on my list.*

One may also choose to set a meaning or purpose for a goal or activity. Example: *I can see I need to change my work situation, so I will set up an appointment with my boss. If that doesn't work, I need to start looking for another job.*

My internal intention may be to choose to see that I need more exercise. Example: *As I leave the house for a walk I set my gaze down the street, roll my shoulders back, and begin walking toward my goal—the end of the block.*

"Someone told me that drishti means to look inward?"

There is often a fine line between looking in and looking out, allowing air and thoughts to flow in and out. Think of *drishti* as an actual eyeball—one can look out or one can look in!

It can also mean to *gaze inward* and ultimately *see* the truth in oneself, or in a particular situation. It can be a very powerful tool for self-examination. Truth and reality can be experienced in many different ways. Sometimes we can *see* the truth, *hear* the truth, *smell* the truth, *touch* the truth, and *feel* or *sense* the truth.

Drishti also encompasses all those *ah-ha insights* that come at unexpected moments—while taking a shower, walking in the woods, talking to a friend or writing in your journal. It can be the simple *insight* of observing that my left shoulder always seems to pull forward in a certain posture, or as complicated as intense therapy involving a child-hood family issue.

Drishti can be the process of looking inward: *Oops, I need to adjust my left shoulder,* or *I need purchase another journal to continue writing about how my childhood issues are affecting me today.* The *drishti* is a powerful tool for creating and increasing your personal pursuit of creating more **Chocolate Yoga** opportunities in your life today.

"So this drishti can be physical and psychological?"

If you think of our eyes as *windows to the soul,* it may be easier to get a sense of *drishti.* It can be used as a tool to *see* the truth.

On a physical level that could be seeing the dishes in the sink or the pile of laundry on your closet floor. Or it may mean seeing that your pants don't fit and they did not shrink in the dryer, you are simply putting on weight around your waist.

The refreshing thing about tuning into your *drishti* is that it can be used as pure information. What you choose to do with the information is always up to you.

"I can SEE the bags under my eyes from not sleeping and I don't need to step on a scale to tell me I am overweight. So how's this going to actually help me right now?"

Drishti is seeing the truth. What stresses are keeping you from sleeping well and why are you overweight? Most of us do not want to go there. We'd rather take a sleeping pill, have a drink, or blame something or someone else. But unless we dig a bit deeper and are willing to see our truth, we will continue to repeat our patterns. The willingness to be honest comes from within and there is no short cut.

"I thought this Chocolate Yoga concept was about pleasure, this self examination stuff sounds pretty painful."

I do not know anyone who is living **Chocolate Yoga** 24/7. All I know is that most of us are dealing with stress in some way, shape or form every day. It may be a minor issue: *What should I eat for lunch?* For some of us that may be a major issue. It's all relative!

I may be stressing on what I should fix for lunch, when suddenly the washing machine starts overflowing or the phone rings with news of a death in the family. Suddenly my priorities and focus are shifted off my lunch decision and onto more pressing issues.

Gazing into the refrigerator, I may acknowledge how lucky I am that

I do have a choice on what to eat, whereas many people do not even know if or when they will eat today.

By using my *drishti* to gaze in and out, I am training myself to put things into perspective. And this in turn is helping me deal with my stress and weight issues in a very realistic manner.

"But the truth hurts!"

Yes and no. Have you ever broken a relationship—with a person, job or situation—that was absolutely toxic for your health and sanity, and felt relief afterwards? As painful as the truth can be, it can also be incredibly liberating. When you finally break free from something or someone who was holding you back, you will find your breathing becoming deeper and smoother. When you can make a healthy decision that has been stressing you for hours, days, weeks or years, you will suddenly find and feel space and peace in your life.

Telling the truth, especially to yourself, is like building a muscle or a good habit. It may be uncomfortable at first—to find the time to exercise or floss, or make a change that you know is ultimately the best for your well-being—but, after a while you will notice that you put up less smoke and mirrors in front of what you really want and are better able to communicate with your true self.

All of the above is in the context of not running around and telling everyone *your* truths, unless it will add to the intimacy and truth of your relationship. Nor does it do much good to tell someone else what *their* truths are, unless it is done with love and you truly believe it will contribute to your relationship.

I am not a therapist, nor would I ever advise anyone to do anything without listening or tuning into their inner *drishti* first. You owe it to yourself to listen to yourself with as much light as possible.

"Why are gazing points so important in practicing and living yoga?"

The gaze can literally help you balance—whether you are brushing your teeth, reaching up to change a light bulb or doing a yoga pose. Stand up. Close your eyes. What happens? Can you balance? Are you dizzy? The balance of the body is very dependent on a steady gaze. The gaze works as an extra set of limbs to support the body in where it wants to go.

Think of your eyes as lasers and sensors extending out into the world picking up all sorts of information for maintaining equilibrium.

Gazing points are also invaluable tools for traveling internally.

Notice the difference when you close your eyes. What do you see? Using your breath in conjunction with your internal and external *drishti* will give you insights into your truth and the reality of a situation.

"The gazing points seems very limited to just body points, how would I apply this concept to my real everyday life?"

There is a beautiful Native American story about how the elders used to train their youth to really look and see the world around them. When the young people would come back from chores, the elders would ask questions about what side of the trees the moss was growing on, or how many animal tracks they noticed. This training was not only for survival of the individual and the tribe, but it increased sensitivity to the environment and one's relationship with nature.

The gaze also can be used as an instant meditation. Notice the sunlight shining through the leaves of a tree, watch a bird looking for worms, or note the tail lights on the vehicles in front of you on the highway. Watch your hands dancing over the computer keyboard, chopping vegetables, or turning the pages of this book. It is all connected. Soften your gaze and sense the world around you.

"Sounds a bit like day dreaming out the window as a kid in school."

There are some similarities in finding a gazing point and day dreaming! They both can produce a feeling of calm and equanimity. Quite often, especially as children, we could relax by looking out a window at clouds, trees and birds. These same natural elements can still work for us today as *drishti* gazing points.

Many spas and meditation centers are located in beautiful natural environments. It is often a challenge to find peacefulness in a more urban setting, but it can be done. One can gaze at a picture of nature, a small plant, a rock nestled in your hands, a tree outside your office window, a photo or postcard of a loved one, holy person, or art piece, a candle or maybe even a cloud in the sky! Notice the next time you are on an airplane, how many people sitting by the window, are just peacefully gazing out the window.

"Are there different kinds of drishti to use when practicing yoga?"

My favorite three gazing points to help me balance are the tip of the nose, the hands (especially the tips of my fingers), and the feet (especially the big toes).

After I set my gaze and breath into the posture, I often can feel a sense of surrender turning into peace. Even if my balance only lasts for a few seconds, gazing points are wonderful tools for creating relaxation within the tension. Your gaze is invaluable for achieving balance, literally and figuratively!

Remember, these gazing points are wonderful to practice wherever you are. Over time you will begin to notice that you do it just naturally without really thinking, *Oh, I'm feeling a bit out of balance, maybe I should find a focus point.* You'll just do it!

"Are there other gazing points?"

The following are classic yoga gazing points written in English and then Sanskrit. You don't need to remember the exact names. We probably played with all these gazing points as children, especially gazing at the tip of our nose trying to go cross-eyed.

These gazing points can be used to focus a wandering mind or assist in balancing, and they can help to relieve tension between the body and the mind. These gazing points may also be used during meditation.

Try them out anytime during your day, especially while performing routine tasks, but **NOT while operating moving vehicles or equipment.**

- The tip of the nose (*Nasagrai drishti*).
- The area between the eyebrows (*Ajna chakra* or *Bhrumadbya* or *Broomadhya drishti*).
- The belly button (*Nabi chakra* or *Nabbi chakra drishti*).
- The hand/hands *(Hastagram* or *Hastagrai drishti).*
- The thumbs (*Angushthamadbyam* or *Angusta ma dyai drishti*).
- The toes (*Padayoragram* or *Padhayoragrai drishti*).
- The owl (*Parshva drishti*): this means gazing toward the far right or the far left—like an owl. This gazing point has the same name for gazing either right or left! The thinking is that if you continue to turn right, you will eventually be facing left!
- Up to the sky (*Urdhva* or *Antara drishti*).

Note: *There are different spellings of the above drishtis depending on what Sanskrit translation you are using or which scholar/yoga teacher you are studying with.*

"I have a yoga teacher who says to never close our eyes during asana practice. Why is that?"

There are different schools of thought on keeping your eyes open during your *asana* (posture) practice or closing your eyes while in certain postures. On a very practical level, by keeping your eyes open and softly gazing at the tip of your nose or your toes, you will notice that it is easier to balance. As soon as you close your eyes, there is that wonderful opportunity to space out and loose the connection with the body. The gazing points are tremendous assistants in keeping your balance.

The next time you have your legs up the wall, close your eyes and see what happens.

It is beneficial to play with the gaze and the gazing points because you will learn to tune into the realities both inside and outside your body and your mind. There is no right or wrong. Experiment as you go about your daily tasks and *asana* practice, and simply note the differences in practicing the postures with your eyes open or closed.

"My best friend said that yoga improved her vision... I find that hard to believe."

There could be several things going on, including the amount of stress your friend has been experiencing. How much time does she spend staring at a computer screen or electronic device? Sometimes just taking frequent eye breaks helps to relax the eyes.

If she is doing some yoga stretches, she may be experiencing increased relaxation in the neck, shoulders and upper body. She may be using her breath to tune in to her body and her mind, and making changes in her life that are improving her vision. I've noticed when I make one small change there is this a subtle (and sometimes not so subtle) *domino effect*, where all sorts of good changes start to happen.

The more you practice breathing mindfully and listening to your body, the more aware you are—you will notice your body telling you what you need to do now, including relaxing the eyes. It is also important to let people *use* yoga to explain phenomena in their lives if it is not causing harm to themselves or anyone else. Everyone's experience is very personal and there is value in honoring their truth.

"I have a hard time focusing in class or practicing at home. I look out the window, stare at the clock, notice people's outfits, or start thinking about preparing my next meal, sometimes I spend the whole class letting my eyes and my mind wander around the room."

Welcome to reality. The mind is a wonderful time travel machine. When I find my mind gazing all over the room, I let it wander. I acknowledge the rain outside the window, the clock, nice leggings on so-and-so, and what I am going to eat as soon as I finish this practice. Then I focus on my breath, and bingo, I am back in my body.

Then my mind starts to wander around again. Like a toddler going exploring. Someone leaves class to go to the bathroom… *hmm, maybe I should go to the bathroom… hmm,* back to the breath…. *hmm.* A few breaths later I am thinking about *a chocolate chip cookie, and Jenny's birthday… have to remember to send a card…. hmm,* back to the breath. So it goes. All these monkeys chattering in my mind sometimes turn into an entire zoo of interesting thoughts, all clamoring for attention.

The more I use my breath, the more I can let go and just let it flow. Sometimes I visualize each monkey thought sitting on its own rubber raft floating down the river navigating the rapids, knowing that I will catch up to them later.

I am learning not to fight my thoughts, and the never-ending *TO DO* list that continues to grow as I sit in relaxation! The more mindfully I breathe throughout my day, the better my life works! And sometimes I even finish some tasks on my to-do list!

"I have no time to do anything. Just listening to all these suggestions is stressing me out."

One of the most challenging people we need to take care of is—ourself. You will find that over time, the more you just take deep breaths, you will create more time for the *right* things to happen in your life. We tend to make everything more complicated than it really needs to be.

You brush your teeth every day, why not take an extra 30 seconds to place a hot washcloth over your eyes and take a deep breath?

You make at least one phone call a day, why not look out the window as you wait and get a minute of instant meditation. You usually make a meal once a day, even take-out food looks better on a tray with real dishes and silverware.

There are so many ways to take care of and feed your eyes. Let the breath be your guide, and you will find more time in your life for very simple and sweet **Chocolate Yoga** moments!

Drishti Techniques for Stress & Weight Management

Ground Rules and Guidelines for Drishti Exercises

Stop, Look, Listen, and Breath. When in doubt—Breathe. Breathe. Breathe. Going deeper? Breathe. Scared? Breathe. Dizzy? Breathe. Shaky? Breathe. Remember to breathe between the stimulus and your response.

Start with where you are now. Honor your body, your injuries, surgeries and memories.

Listen to your body/mind—pain is the messenger. If you experience any sharp pains, back off—this includes emotional pain. Take a deep breath and reassess the situation.

There is no rush. You have all the time in the world. By backing off and gently working with your body, you will go deeper.

Have fun, experiment, lighten up, and smile. It actually helps with creating eye health!

#1. Clock Face

I like to do this eye exercise as slowly as I can, and if I have time, two times in each direction is really delicious. This is an excellent stretch to do when taking an *eye break* from staring at a computer, television or movie screen. It's also good to do after sitting through long meetings, lectures or trainings. This exercise offers great eye relief.

- Sit up as straight as you can in a chair, on the floor, or seated leaning against the wall. Find a comfortable place to rest your hands.
- Take off your glasses. If you are wearing contacts, be mindful of your comfort level.
- Close your eyes and take a deep breath, and then slowly open your eyes keeping them slightly open and soft.
- Slowly raise your eyeballs to stretch up to 12 o'clock. Then, as slowly as you can, make your way around an imaginary clock face to 1, 2, and stretching far right to 3, 4, 5. Continue stretching far down to 6, then over to 7, 8, and far left to 9. Stretch on up to 10, 11, then finally back to 12 o'clock.
- Take a deep breath and repeat by shifting your eyes counter-clockwise from 12, 11, 10, 9, 8, 7, 6, 5, 4, 3, 2, 1 and back to 12.
- Do both sides and remember to take your time.

#2. Warm Hands Mini Spa

This exercise is great to do anytime you need to bring warmth and relaxation to your face. Start with clean hands. This simple exercise can be done sitting or lying down on your back.

- Take your glasses off, or if you are wearing contacts be mindful of applying very gentle pressure to the eye area.
- Bring the palms of your hands together and vigorously rub them together until your hands become really warm.
- They may even begin to get hot.
- Slowly release your hands, close your eyes and then cover them, gently making your hands into two soft eye cups. Rest your finger tips on your forehead, and the heels of your hands on your cheeks. Make sure there is no direct pressure on your eyes—the palms of your hands are cupped to make a little hollow. Exert absolutely NO pressure on the eye balls.
- Let your eyes soften and roll gently backwards in their sockets.
- Feel your warm finger tips soothing away any winkles, frown lines, or worries.
- Let the palms of your hands rest gently on your cheeks.
- Let your facial muscles slowly soften and relax.
- Keep your elbows pointed down, so that there no tension trying to hold your arms up.
- As your hands cool down, keep your eyes closed as you slowly release your hands into your lap with your palms facing up.

Sit or lie quietly for a few breaths, enjoying that sense of peace and tranquility. When you are ready, slowly open your eyes and enjoy the rest of your day.

#3. Hand *Mudras*

Our hands can be used as *drishti* focus tools for stress and weight management.

One of my heroes is Helen Keller. As a child I read everything I could about her. I was fascinated with the concept of blindness and how one could be so alive, yet not be able to *see*. How did she know what food to eat? What if someone gave her a dead cockroach and told her it was a piece of candy? How did she survive and thrive without seeing or hearing? It took me years to realize that one can *see* through any or all of the senses. The brain is an amazing processor that connects us to our senses and ultimately our heart.

The yogis believe that our arms are extensions of our hearts. Hence our hands are connected to our hearts. This sense of touch is invaluable in helping babies thrive, comforting people in an emotional situation, or simply reaching out to someone, looking deep into their eyes and shaking their hand. Have you ever had the experience of looking deep into someone's eyes and felt that ZING of a connection? It may have been a complete stranger walking along, a lover, or even *locking eyes* with someone over the dinner table as you shared a mutual joke.

Our hands may be used as personal stress and weight management tools. They can be your *drishti* touch stones, to help you connect your heart and brain. Watch your hands as you are preparing your snacks or meals. Slow down and observe the knife cutting. See what happens when you totally focus on the task at hand, do not talk on the phone, listen to the news or think of anything else. Just chop, cut, stir, set the table—whatever you are doing—observe. We are rarely **in the moment,** so it may be helpful to talk out loud as if you were doing a monologue, *wow, look at these lovely apples, hmmm, funny slice mark on the side, maybe it got nicked in transit... look at this pattern, looks like a super nova from the side... wonder if I cut them thinner if they would taste differently.*

You get the idea, seems kind of silly, but it is a very powerful exercise for being in the moment. Meal preps can become instant meditation and can also help you *see* how often we are not in the moment. We think it's educational to talk to toddlers and children with enthusiasm about food preparation and eating. We explain how things are grown, harvested, packaged; then we cut a pear and look at patterns, or make funny faces on our peanut butter sandwiches. What happened to playing with our food? Talking to our food? Eating half a sandwich (in half an hour), then running off to play? We forgot how to tune into our inner reality, which may be not to finish everything on our plate, or to be adult enough to not take so much in the first place! Some of our obesity comes from not paying attention to our inner and outer reality. We tune out. Shut down. And stuff our face.

I grew up in a big family and we all rotated through making dinner. One night in high school I had read about an *Esalen Institute* eating exercise. I surprised my family by making a big spaghetti dinner, and set the table with no utensils and lots of napkins. The idea was to eat with our hands. After all the protest died down and my elegant mother began eating spaghetti with her hands, we all got into it. We finished dinner with a big iced chocolate cake, which we demolished with tons of laughter and giggles. It is now part of the official collection of funny family stories. It also taught me an important lesson in connecting my hands with reality. And to this day, when I am dining alone, I often eat my meal with my hands and it tastes exceptionally good—try it! For extra credit, close your eyes, and see what happens!

There is also the idea of *grace*. Bowing our head before eating, usually with our hands in a prayer position, and expressing our gratitude for the food we are about to eat. Many of us do not do this, except under the social pressure of a holiday, special occasion or a meal with family/ friends who 'do grace'. And yet there is something to be said for slowing down and using our hands to express what is in our hearts.

There are entire books written on hand positions or gestures *(mudras)*. We all recognize the basic international communication hand gestures of waving hello, goodbye, stop, or the middle finger raised usually expressing displeasure. The classic prayer position of pressing the palms of the hands together, usually with the head tipped slightly toward the chest is a timeless gesture that crosses all cultures since the beginning of civilization. This gesture has been depicted in paintings, wall and temple carvings, statues, frescos, sculptures, icons and photographs. This gesture is repeated daily around the world as people press their hands together in greeting, prayer, blessings, grace or meditation.

When you begin to think of your hands extending energy or creating circuits of energy—as you press them together or touch one finger to another—you will begin to feel and sense your *prana* (breath as energy) flowing. The following *mudras* are helpful tools in managing your stress and weight issues.

- *Namaste/prayer:* There are several translations of word *Namaste*. *Nam* means bow, *as* means I, and *te* means you—as in, "I bow to you." The word is usually linked with placing your hands together, palms lightly touching in a prayer position with your thumbs gently resting between your breasts at your heart center. This position is extremely comforting. One may choose to tip your head towards your fingertips. Keep your eyes soft as you gaze down at your fingertips or close your eyes. This hand position is often used when greeting another person as in, *hello, goodbye, nice to see you,* or simply *thank you!* It is often used in yoga classes to open and close the practice with honor, respect and acknowledgement.
- *Yogi Wisdom:* Sitting cross-legged, extend your arms out to the side so that your hands are resting on your knees with the palms facing up. Don't worry if your hands are resting on your thighs, it is more important to be comfortable so that you can breathe.
  - Bring your thumb and the first finger of your hand together so they are lightly touching. You'll notice that your fingers are making a circle, like the hand signal OK.
  - Roll your shoulders down and away from your ears; soften the face, especially the jaw and the mouth as you drop your chin gently down toward your collarbone *(Jalandhara Bandha)*.
  - If you feel any discomfort, be sure to wiggle and do what you need to do to get comfortable in this classic meditation pose. Continue breathing deeply as you extend your inhales and your exhales.
  - There are many options here—listening to your breath, listening to music, practicing one of the breathing meditations outlined in the previous sections, reciting your favorite prayer or chanting your personal mantra.
- *Palms Facing Up:* Follow the Yogi Wisdom instructions above, but instead of bringing the thumb and the first finger together, let the back of your hands rest on your knees or on your thighs with your palms facing up. The fingers will naturally curl slightly upward. This is a very strong open-heart pose. It also represents being vulnerable and exposed. If thoughts tend to pop into your mind, you may want to keep your journal nearby to record insights, or have a piece of paper to jot down a few words

to trigger your memory later. As with all of yoga, remember to keep the breath flowing and ease into and out of every posture, including moving your hands slowly and mindfully.

- **Palms Facing Down:** This is very similar to the *mudra* above, except that the hands are resting palms facing down on the knees or the thighs. Remember to roll your shoulders back and down away from your ears. Leaning against the wall will give you extra support along the spine and is a good reminder to move your breath *up* and *down* the spine. You'll be able to feel the back of the lungs expanding as the diaphragm lifts and contracts. Sometimes it feels good to send the breath up and down your arms and your legs, giving yourself an *internal massage,* to increase that feeling of serenity.

- **Hands in Lap:** Place the right hand on top of the left hand with both palms facing upward. This classic *mudra* is depicted in many statues of Buddha, sitting up straight and tall, with his hands in his lap, right hand on top of the left with the palms facing up. You often see a flower or offering resting in the cradle of the right palm. You may choose to place a flower, smooth rock or any object that has a special meaning to you, directly in front of you or in the palm of your hand. These symbols will often become powerful focus or *drishti* tools in your meditation practice. The head is usually tilted forward by dropping the chin toward the collarbone. Your eyes may be open or closed. This pose is incredibly meditative and relaxing.

Note: *Sometimes my hands know exactly what position feels right today. At other times, if I am distracted or out of sorts I will do all of the above hand postures—just holding each position for a breath or two before moving on to the next one. By the end of the sequence, I know exactly which one is the one I need. Sometimes I go for weeks preferring one hand position over all the other options. Then suddenly I need to try something different. I haven't figured out a pattern, I have just learned to trust the process.*

⚭

#4. The Reality Journal

To really *see* what is going on in one's own life is a very difficult task. Yet the only way to make real change is to honestly question ourselves. We are often full of drama, stomping our feet—usually around the theme, "Life would be so much better if I wasn't so stressed about...". Fill in the blank with everything from my weight, my spouse, my job, my in-laws, the neighbors, the war, the price of gas, my messy house, more bills, health insurance, car repairs... you get the idea.

Most of us have at least one stressor that we can name right now. I haven't found a way to skip this part of life. I have only learned what works for me. And the big question behind all the stressors in our life is, **What is really going on in my life?**

Notice the next time you get irritated with someone—it is usually not the person—it is the situation. We are constantly mirroring our truth, whether we like it or not. We fall into patterns and habits, and until we examine our truth under the light we will not be able to change and go in a healthier direction.

Start writing, singing or talking. This is one of the most powerful stress and weight management tools ever. Start wherever you are and don't stop. The process of venting on paper in priceless. You will be able to see yourself and deal with your truth. I write in my journal almost every day, and it is not always pretty. I joke that if anyone ever read my journal, I could easily be put away in a facility. So yes, many pages are shredded every year; however, I know that I have purged onto the paper many thoughts that I would have swallowed and probably tried to bury under tons of cookies.

I look at the journal process being as important as bathing, brushing and flossing. It is preventive medicine for my mental health. It is also an ancient yogi thought that the arms are connected to the heart—so when you reach out to hug someone that energy is going toward your heart. I like to think that my hands writing are connecting me with my heart, and getting me out of my chattering *story-creating* head and re-connecting me to the truth in my heart.

What's really going on in my life?

- **Keep a journal.** It is one of the most simple, yet powerful self-examination tools.
  - It does not have to be fancy, any simple notebook will work.
  - The most important element of journaling is to tell the truth.
  - Writing your thoughts, feelings, and situations will offer invaluable opportunities to gain insight into your reality. It is not helpful to judge, just write the truth and you will begin to observe the patterns that keep you **weighed** down.
  - By telling the truth, you can start to let go and release what isn't working for you and begin to move toward creating a healthier more balanced life.
- **Write or draw** something every day.
- **Write a poem.** It doesn't have to rhyme, be perfect or make sense.
- **Write a letter** to yourself, family member or friend if you are having a hard time getting started.
  - You may want to write to someone or *something* that you currently have issues with, it can even be to someone who has died or is famous, whether you've met them or not. The point is to start the dialog and follow the path wherever it may lead you in the moment.
- **Choosing a word or image** is another way to get started (e.g., truth, beauty, health, food, money, thighs, things I would like to do before I die), and start writing.
- **Ask yourself a question.** *If I could wave a magic wand what would I change? If I won the sweepstakes what would I do? Is there any way to start living the life I always wanted? What do I need to do next in my life?*
- **List whatever is stressing you today.** Circle the stressors that you can do something about right now (e.g., my next meal). Cross out the stressors that you have no control over (e.g., the weather). And draw a wiggly line through whatever stresses are NOT yours, but you've taken them on for whatever reason (e.g., your spouse's boss; your best friend's infertility; your son's girl friend dumps him; your step-mother's alcoholism). Find a healthy way to support your loved ones without taking on their pain.
  - Sing: *Row, row, row your boat gently down the stream…* Remember to row YOUR boat down the stream. Unless you are invited into someone's boat to help them row—and accept the responsibility—stay in your own boat and keep rowing!

- **The Gratitude Journal.** Before you go to sleep or just after you wake up, take a few minutes to write down five things that you are grateful for today. You may also choose to draw them or write a poem. Loosen up. Be creative. On your birthday see if you can come up with a list to match your birthday number.
- **What do you need to do before you die?** Your physician has just informed you that you have a rare disease and that you will die within one year. How will you live this final year? And why not start living that life right now?
  - Another version of the above is that you have only 24 hours to live. What do you need to do before you die? This could include any unfinished business including (but not limited to), contacting those people who you really love and honor to thank them for being part of your life, and/or those people you need to ask forgiveness for any past transgressions or unfulfilled responsibilities. Imagine the lightness and freedom you will feel as you deal with the unfinished business in your life.
- **Write just the facts, no feelings.** Can you write an accident or an incident report? Just state the facts as in a police or medical report, without the dramatic interpretation.
- **Write just your feelings, no facts.** Rant, rave and be as crazy as your dare. You may choose to shred this one.

Remember, as in the practice of yoga postures, your journal is a tool, a guide for communicating with your truth. If you have any fears about someone finding your journal and using it against you, you may want to hide it, shred it, or look boldly at the situation and examine your relationship with that person.

The more you begin to tell the truth the easier it will be to live your truth. You'll be surprised how much better you will feel.

You also will be surprised how often the answer to a problem or situation will just flow from your fingertips. Sometimes we get so wrapped up in our stories that we cannot SEE the truth—the *drishti* within!

❦

#5. The *Drishti* of Weight Management

Name that Focus

Have you ever found yourself grazing around the kitchen eating everything in sight whether it is just before dinner, after dinner or nowhere near a meal time? Why are you in the kitchen? What are you looking for? It is sometimes referred to in the literature as *mindless eating, noshing with no end in sight,* or *going unconscious.* Needless to say, it is usually totally annoying. And you can stop it by practicing a *drishti* technique called **Name That Focus!**

This *drishti* exercise came out of a religion class that I took years ago and has been a priceless technique to help me create instant mindfulness. Have you ever found yourself driving to work so wrapped up in some drama that is unfolding in your life that suddenly you are in the employee parking lot, not even aware of how you got there? When I find my mind wandering all around my world of concerns, problems and situations, I am not paying attention to what is going on in the moment. I take a really deep breath and literally focus on what is right in front of me.

Driving Mindfully

I am driving, thinking about other things, not really paying attention to the reality outside my window. When I catch my mind wandering, I take a deep inhale and then exhale. As I begin to notice and focus on exactly what is happening outside—**I name it.** So my dialog may go something like this:

Oh, look at that cute yellow Volkswagen on the right… Garbage truck pulling out, slow down… Pedestrian coming up on the left, talking on the phone… looks like the city trimmed those trees, I don't remember seeing that roof top from here. Wow… lots of people at the bus stop better slow down… must be a school near here… yup… speed limit is 25.

I have reframed my sometimes irritating drive to work as an opportunity to do my *Driving Mindfully* meditation. Not only do I arrive fully present, but I have fed my mind with interesting observations.

Chopping Carrots

My mind usually wanders all over the place—either ruminating about past actions, non-actions, or worried about future events. When I get in touch with the endless dribble, I can call myself to task by simply asking myself:

What are you doing? I'm chopping carrots... hmm, this one has an interesting pattern... I wonder where these carrots where grown... I think I'll chop them into several different shapes for variety... wow, these are juicy... my knife is turning orange... this one is really funny looking.

And then I just listen to my inhales and my exhales, reminding myself that chopping carrots can be a wonderful meditation opportunity!

Just the Facts

I have a habit of story telling, which usually drives the male species in my family nuts, especially when they just want me to just cut to the chase. That's why I call this one *Just the Facts*. I try to be aware of the difference between the story telling and just telling the facts as in who, what, where, how, and why. My internal dialog may be something along these lines:

I have to tell Bob that I wasn't able to book the flight that he wanted with his air miles because he would have to change planes twice, but the really nice agent suggested that we move the departure date to mid-week, but I knew that wouldn't work if your sister picking you up at the airport, remember that's the airport with the rent-a-car station three miles from the main terminal. So I went on-line and checked two other airlines. The first one had only one stop but the wait time would have been four hours and the second airline only had a twenty minute window between arrival and departure, which I know is just cutting it too close, especially running through an airport with your knee not up to par, so I called your sister, and her best friend will pick you up if need be, then I called the really nice airline agent back and of course got a real grumpy one. You get the picture.

What Bob wants to hear is: *I booked a flight for you next Wednesday, with a great connection and a good rent-a-car deal. Here is a print out with all the information including your confirmation numbers for the airline and rent-a-car.*

Sometimes it is better to cut to the chase, do the facts really need a story? Well, sometimes yes, and sometimes no. Be mindful of the recipient of the information, do they need just the facts, or do they need to hear the story?

How much drama do we need surrounding our food choices? Does the listener need to hear all about the battle between the donut and the carrot? Maybe yes and maybe no!

I often have a very difficult time going out to eat with people or at a party, when someone goes into a long soliloquy on variations of: *I really shouldn't be eating this... I know it's really bad for me... but since I worked out this morning I really deserve this treat...* or *I know I will pay for this later when I step on the scale tomorrow.*

How much time is spent on making food/eating decisions? If you stopped fussing about every morsel of food, what would you be doing with all that extra time?

If you really need a dialog, you may want to take it to your journal or go to the bathroom and talk to the mirror. Or if you are with like-minded people, you may want to ask someone to listen and help you hear your true issues. If not, please try to figure out what you really need or want. It is also OK to share the treat in question, and/or take some home for later. That way everyone wins and you can get on with living your life.

Really Listening

The challenge here is to really listen. To be able to listen to the speaker and actually hear what they are saying is an art and skill that grows with practice. My problem is that I rarely listen without jumping in to interrupt. I finish people's thoughts and sentences, and often offer a solution that does not work for the speaker. This ultimately creates more stress and tension, instead of increasing resolution and peace.

If I really listen, then I will inevitably pick up several layers and be able to filter and hear more than just the words. I become an *active listener,* and may ultimately lower everyone's stress levels.

The next time someone speaks to you, notice where you go while they are talking. This technique also works on listening to yourself! See if you can really hear what you are saying when you are talking with someone. Or if you are by yourself and have privacy, talk to yourself. See *(drishti)* if you can really listen to the truth behind your words.

If you are going to have a cookie, have a cookie.

Remember the tag line from the cookie ad a few years ago, *"If you're going to have a cookie, have a cookie,"* with a big chocolate chip cookie taking up the entire page?

I love that concept. It is total mindfulness. So if you are going to have a cookie: ***get the exact right cookie!*** Why are we eating the whole box of cookies? Why can't we find that perfect cookie? Why aren't we satisfied with just one cookie?

Because we are looking for something else. And the key to weight management is identifying our stressors as different from our actual needs and wants. We get mixed up in the stories, the multi-tasking, and the to-do list, without ever sitting down with the truth. *Do I need a cookie? Do I want a cookie? Do I need a hug? Do I need to scream?* What's really going on here?

Stop multi-tasking everything. Notice what happens when you do just one thing at a time. This is the *drishti* in mindfulness. We actually increase our stress levels by trying to focus on multiple activities and tasks. The gaze and the mind cannot be everywhere at once. Why do we think that we can do it all? Why not do one thing at a time. See what happens to your stress level. See what happens to your weight.

Gratitude

I sometimes call this the *thank you thank you thank you* meditation. I always feel so much better after practicing this—even if only for 30 seconds! This simple awareness exercise will bring much joy into your day and your life. It is a wonderful grounding form of meditation to do when you are feeling out of sorts, depressed or unfocused. It is very simple and powerful. For everything you do and touch—give thanks.

Slow down. As you brush your teeth, thank the running warm water, your wonderful toothbrush, great tasting toothpaste, the knowledge that flossing is helping your entire cardiovascular system. Thank your clothes and your shoes. As you fill the tea kettle, thank the people who made it. Maybe it was a wedding present or belonged to your mother, say thank you. Mentally say thank you for the gift of boiling water. Thank your favorite tea cup or mug and the tea leaves. You are acknowledging their presence in your life. As you get into your car to drive to work, thank the people who worked hard to bring you that vehicle. I am sure you see where this is going.

In less than five minutes you can put your mind and body into a beautiful place of gratitude. It is even more powerful when you stop and thank the person in front of you for their smile, assisting you in the grocery checkout lane, the mail delivery person, the person who stops their car to let you walk across the street, the neighbor who always waves a cheery hello... the list is endless and the joy is boundless.

The *drishti* of weight management is a lifetime practice of really truly being able to **see** your truth.

Can you name that focus? What are you focused on right now? Are you reading? Are you thinking about what is for dinner? Are you breathing? See what happens when you begin to name that focus—whether you are driving, chopping carrots, stating the facts without the drama, really listening to yourself and others, thanking everything and everyone in your world including that one single perfect cookie!

Questions to Ask Myself

*What am I pretending not to **see** right now?*

Place your hand on your heart and ask yourself:
What truth am I hiding from?

Who or what can I thank right now for being in my
life?

What can I let go of right now?

The most beautiful things
in the world cannot be seen
with the eyes,
but only with the human heart.

~ Helen Keller

... Meditation in Motion ...

walking swimming eating golfing reading sleeping running cleaning showering sailing skating skiing laughing driving soccer basketball baseball dancing diving shopping knitting sewing gardening singing working biking laundry camping hiking jogging tai chi tennis fishing surfing drawing horseback riding skateboarding sledding drawing painting writing gaming playing acting teaching being jumping gymnastics

... Breathe ...

walking swimming eating golfing reading sleeping running cleaning showering sailing skating skiing laughing driving soccer basketball baseball dancing diving shopping knitting sewing gardening singing working biking laundry camping hiking jogging tai chi tennis fishing surfing drawing horseback riding skateboarding sledding drawing painting writing gaming playing acting teaching being jumping gymnastics

... Just Breathe ...

Chapter 4

Asanas

The Postures:
Meditation in Motion

Questions I've Been Asked

"What are asanas?"

Asana is the Sanskrit word for a yoga *posture*. The literal translation is *a comfortable seat*, e.g., *a posture that eases the body and the mind*. These physical poses where originally developed over the past 5,000 years to simply quiet the mind and get your body ready to meditate.

Technically any posture that you are engaged in can be called an *asana*. So there is the walking *asana*, the brushing teeth *asana*, the playing tennis *asana*, or the driving *asana*. The list is endless. The postures are a tool to bring awareness into your life through your body, whether in stillness or in motion.

"I've only taken one yoga class and it was horrible. The teacher used Sanskrit names for all the poses and everyone was skinny and flexible. I never went back."

Practicing yoga *asanas* in a group situation can be intimidating and inspiring. There is always someone in every group that is smarter, prettier and more flexible than we are. That is reality of comparisons, but does it really matter? Keep trying different classes, styles and teachers until you find something that resonates with you.

It doesn't matter where you are in your physical life-cycle, there are yoga poses for *every* body. We all need to begin our practice within the reality of our *current* physical body. This includes acknowledging our physical limitations including injuries, surgeries and stress levels. The postures presented in this book are simple and straightforward, yet they offer variations that will keep you challenged for a lifetime.

"The yoga postures taught in yoga studios and on DVDs seem too complicated."

Sometimes just standing up straight and tall can be construed as *complicated*. It is probably a combination of creativity and human nature to push the envelope—in this case to bend, twist and rotate the physical body to see what happens! The yoga postures are just a way to play with the body. There are approximately 84 basic *asana* postures and over 840,000 variations.

Most yoga practitioners have their favorite postures and least favorite or more challenging postures. Longtime practitioners will tell you how their practice has changed over time, and that often the *easy* postures become more difficult and the challenging postures become easier. Even if you are practicing the same postures daily, they will be different because we change on a daily basis.

The most important element is your attitude of just trying to move your body in different ways and using your gaze (*drishti*) to observe yourself. If you breathe mindfully and go only as far as you can go in the moment, you will have truly arrived at listening to your true self. The postures are as complicated as you make them.

"I find myself always holding my breath as I go in and out of postures, my teachers are always telling me to breathe. Why am I holding my breath?"

I would be curious to see if you are holding your breath as you go about doing other activities in your life. Notice if *not* breathing is situational. Sometimes I find myself holding my breath when I have to deal with people I don't like, or I need to do something new, or I am walking into a room full of people I don't know.

Observe yourself in action and non-action. As you learn to use the breath to move in and out of postures and situations, you will find yourself feeling more balanced and confident. New situations often become creative challenges, instead of something to avoid and dread. Using your breath mindfully in many situations will help to build up your stamina. Breathing mindfully is the key to everything that you will do in your lifetime.

"I don't have time to practice yoga or go to a class, what can I do?"

There are so many ways to do the postures (*asanas*) that you will surprise yourself with your creativity. Look for opportunities to breathe mindfully wherever you are, doing whatever you are doing. The postures in this book can be done anywhere and at anytime. If you can find 3 to 5 minutes a day to put your legs up the wall, you've made a great start and may even find other opportunities throughout the day to squeeze in a mini *asana*!

You may also notice that the more you practice breathing and being mindful, the less stress you will hold on to. You may be tired at the end of the day, but it will be a pleasurable tiredness, as in a long energizing nature walk where your body, mind and spirit have soaked up energy and released energy. You will be experiencing that wonderful feeling of equilibrium and a feeling that *all is well*.

You will find yourself sleeping better and waking up refreshed, just by coordinating your breath with your movements throughout the day. As your energy levels expand you will find more time to do those things that you really want to do, including having more time to practice yoga postures!

"So many people just do the yoga postures (asanas) and say they are doing yoga. Isn't yoga more that just postures?"

Yes, but we need to start somewhere. Many people all over the world have discovered the gifts of yoga through their body, beginning with practicing classic yoga postures. It is very hard to *not* get more from yoga than just physical benefits—the postures have the ability to slowly seduce you into going deeper. Some people take one class and leave. They never come back. Often they don't like the teacher, the heat, the room, the style—something does not click. Or it is such a big click, it's too scary and they back off entirely.

Others become born again yogis, taking three classes a day and proclaiming that yoga cures everything. Some people may drift in and out of practicing yoga postures for years.

It's okay. Do what works for you. The joy of practicing the yoga postures is that they will definitely take you deeper in a very natural and organic way. There is absolutely no rush.

"Why do I sometimes feel like crying when I am in certain yoga postures? The other day I had my legs up the wall and the tears just started flowing. What's going on?"

Sometimes the combination of the breath and the body in a certain posture will release physical and/or emotional pain, tensions, knots, blocks or resistance. Have you ever had a bad day and someone sincerely asks, "How are you?", and you just start crying? Or sometimes a genuine hug from a dear friend will trigger some tears.

I am not a scientist, physician or therapist; however, I do know from my personal experience as a student and a teacher, as long as the release feels good, it is beneficial. I have also received the most amazing insight into situations or problems I have been wrestling with—like the *ah-ha* flashes one sometimes gets in the shower, on a long walk or talk, or in a dream. When we physically relax, insight bubbles are often allowed to rise to the top of our consciousness, and we are blessed with an answer. Listen to your truth and let the tears wash away whatever needs to be released.

"How do I know how fast or slow to do a posture?"

The greatest thing about the yoga postures is their elasticity. Any posture can be done very slowly, very quickly or somewhere in between. You can hold these postures for as long as you choose. If you are really concentrating on the breathing, and let the breath be your guide you will experience your body in a whole new way. You will also learn to read your body/mind, and be able to pace yourself appropriately.

If you are feeling a bit down or depressed, you may find yourself seeking more movement internally or externally. If you are feeling scattered or have so much to do that you don't know where to begin, you may find yourself seeking a slower pace.

The most wonderful thing about accessing these yoga postures is that you will learn to pace and balance yourself. Think of the postures as self-medication, and use them often to energize and recharge your batteries.

"I get discouraged trying so hard to do these postures, how can I have a better attitude?"

The postures are sometimes challenging no matter what age, weight or physical condition you are in. This includes dealing with a temporary or a chronic health issue, or a personal trauma. Just notice how you deal with the challenge of these postures and how you deal with challenges in your everyday life. Are there similarities? Use the postures to help yourself to live more fully in the present moment. They are powerful teachers, when one begins to listen.

"Some people seem so healthy, what is their secret?"

There are many variations of **breathing, core strength, focus, body movement,** and **relaxation**. You will notice that people who are healthy are practicing these five yoga techniques in one form or another.

Many fitness practitioners claim that they reap all the benefits in their favorite activity. It may be through dancing, golf, walking, tennis, bicycling, swimming, gardening, kayaking, skiing, snowboarding, jogging, running, martial arts, *tai chi*, weight lifting, sailing, singing, or rowing. The activity is not as important as the result of energizing your body, mind and spirit.

If you ask people that you admire for their trade secrets for maintaining a healthy lifestyle, many will share their trials and tribulations for staying physically, mentally, emotionally and spiritually healthy.

You will begin to notice a pattern that involves not only their physical activities, but a deep focus and connection with their family, work, church or community organization. It may be a social or environmental cause, a hobby, a grandchild, being a volunteer, their career or their role as the primary breadwinner.

In other words they have a *passion*. They all have a very clear and motivating reason to get up in the morning and get going. These individuals also rest and/or relax in very personal ways. Most take cat naps, or unabashedly tell you how much sleep they need each night or how little! The point is that they know what they need, how much they need and they get it. They also have activities which absolutely relax them. A high-powered attorney reads romance novels, a gym teacher knits, a bus driver plays miniature golf, a computer programmer gardens, and a full time soccer mom plays the *Sims* online.

Ask. Connect. Do some research and keep exploring. There are many paths up the mountain of life.

"This Legs Up the Wall posture seems so easy, is it really yoga?"

Legs Up the Wall actually is a yoga pose and sometimes goes by its Sanskrit name, *Viparita Karani*. The irony of this simple posture is that it is extremely powerful. The wall is totally supporting your body—there is nowhere you have to go, nothing you have to do. The luxury of just hanging out with your legs up the wall is priceless.

My experience has been and continues to be that this is an *ah-ha* posture. It lends itself to total bliss as the body relaxes and connects with the mind. I often get incredible insights into something that is bothering me. Or I remember to do something as simple as send a birthday card or as intense as a childhood memory that explains my behavior today. Sometimes I grab a quick meditative nap. Sometimes I feel as if I am seeing a therapist—*The Wall!* I have never had any regrets about taking a few minutes to put my legs up the wall.

It's a great transition posture when you are out of sorts and find yourself going on automatic pilot toward donuts, cigarettes or a drug of choice.

It is so much easier to live fully in the moment when one is connected and balanced. All of yoga is seeking to enhance the relationship between the body and the mind so the spirit can thrive.

"What if my spouse or one of my children walks in and sees me lying on the floor with my legs up the wall?"

Invite them to join you. It's a great place to hang out and just rest, talk, re-connect. Most children and teenagers really enjoy this pose and often they will open up and tell you what is on their mind. Create a ritual, your children may even ask to do this posture with you!

This posture may be done in solitude or it can be social. It's okay to talk, laugh, commiserate and share stories. It's a nice way to connect with someone. If you have a dog or a cat, they might just snuggle up next to you!

"I know I need to do this pose, I always feel better afterward, but I keep making up excuses?"

You are not alone. The most common blocks of resistance I have heard people say, including myself are: *I am too tired. I don't have time. Today is not a good day; maybe tomorrow will be better. I'm too emotional to do anything today. I don't have a good space to put my feet up a wall. I'm too fat. I think I'll wait until I drop a few pounds. I really think I need that piece of cake in the fridge right now or else I will die.*

And my answer to myself and everyone else is: ***Take a 3 to 5 minute break right now and put your legs up the wall. And see what happens!***

Body Postures for Stress & Weight Management

Important Note Before Starting The Wall Series

- Make sure that you are leaning against a clear wall, without hanging pictures, mirrors or anything that could fall on you.
- If you are doing the postures leaning against a door, make sure that it is locked or that you won't get interrupted.
- If you are on a bare floor, be sure that the area is sufficiently well padded with a rug, a foam pad or a yoga/exercise mat. Be sure that nothing will slide or be unstable as you do your postures.
- You may have to add padding to a carpeted floor. Again, if the floor surface is too hard be sure to add a mat, thick towel, or small rug. It is very important you are physically very comfortable and well supported while doing any of these wall postures.
- If *Legs Up the Wall* is too uncomfortable, try the *Hassock Asana*, which supports your lower legs. It is a variation of *Legs Up the Wall* and is just as potent.

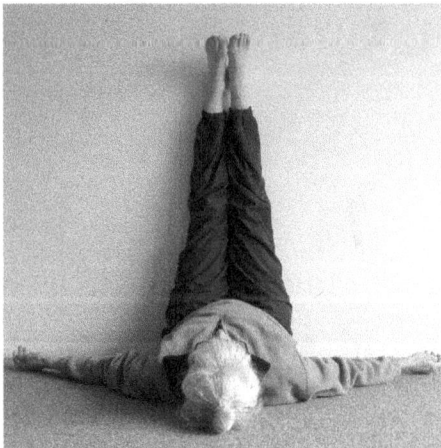

❦

#1. Legs Up the Wall—*Viparita Karani*

How to get into this posture.

- Sit on the floor with your right or left hip against the wall.
- Roll onto your back and wiggle your buttocks until they are as close to the wall as possible.
- Slowly raise your legs so that they are resting on the wall.
- Make sure that there is little or no space between your buttocks and the wall. Your body will look like a letter "L" from the side.
  - If this is uncomfortable, you may experiment with folding a firm blanket under your buttocks. Or you may bend your knees until you feel comfortable. If your hamstrings are really tight, keep your legs bent. Your body will relax over time.
- You may want to begin with just 30 seconds to one minute a day and slowly ease into the posture. Remember at all times that your breath is your guide, if you feel any pain, please back off immediately and consult a trained yoga teacher. This is a lifetime practice, so take your time.
- Move mindfully and slowly always using your inhales and exhales to guide your body.
- Remember to slowly roll out of the posture at any time, especially if you are experiencing any discomfort.

If this is still uncomfortable you may choose to set up a round bolster or several blankets approximately 10 inches from the wall, leaving enough room for your buttocks to rest on the floor and your spine to rest on the bolster/blanket prop. It is very important to AVOID experiencing any sharp pains.

Note: *If after some experimenting and adjusting this simply is NOT working for you. PLEASE STOP and consult a yoga teacher or physical therapist. They will be able to assist you in finding a way to work into this posture.*

Some people have found very creative ways to use couches, padded recliners or their beds to work into this posture (see *Hassock Asana*).

If you would like to stretch into the postures a little bit deeper, or your feet are cold, please keep your socks on. You may find that the fabric slides down the wall and actually accelerates the stretch. Just be careful not to over-stretch or strain your groin area in any of the postures.

As you relax into each posture, always ask your body, *Am I comfortable? Am I so comfortable that I could fall asleep in this posture?*

If not, try something different. You may need to back off or shift your weight. See if you can experiment gently until you find that perfect *ah-ha* moment.

This is an excellent time to listen to soft music or a relaxation/visualization CD/DVD. Sometimes using an eye bag, washcloth, or towel over the eyes may gently induce a sense of relaxation. Or simply place your hands on your tummy and tune in to your inhales and exhales. Always be mindful to go in and out of each posture variation by using the breath to move your body.

✧

#2. Variations of *Viparita Karani:* Legs Up the Wall Posture

Follow the directions above for *Legs Up the Wall.* As soon as you are comfortable, experiment with the following variations. They are all excellent stress reducers, because *the wall does most of the work.* Your job is to hang out and simply breathe!

Sometimes I will just go through the following body position options and then go back and spend more time just relaxing into whatever feels good today.

- Place your hands palms facing down gently resting on your belly. Feel your belly rise and fall like ocean waves with each inhale and exhale.
- Rest your arms firmly on the floor at your sides with your palms facing up or down about 6–12 inches away from your hips. Take a few deep inhales and exhales before moving on.
- Keep your arms on the floor as you slide your arms along the floor until they are above your head. Palms may be facing up or you may want to bend your arms and clasp the outside of your elbows with opposite hands.
  - Move very slowly and mindfully, especially if you have had any shoulder injuries or surgeries. If you experience any sharp

pains, back off immediately and find a more comfortable resting place for your arms.

- Sometimes I like to do *snow angels*. Start by resting your arms on the floor about 6–12 inches from your hips, palms facing up. Then slowly slide them along the floor until they are up over your head.
- If this feels good, you may want to try coordinating your breath with the motion of your arms, inhaling up over your head, pausing as your hands touch, then slowly exhaling as the arms come down to rest along the side of your body.
  - Remember that your hands do NOT have to touch, the idea here is to breathe with the happy childhood memory of making angel shapes in the snow.

Sometimes I leave my legs straight up the wall, and other times they are in an open "V" position. This is an excellent stress reducer, because the wall is totally supporting your legs. Your job is to simply enjoy and breathe!

- You may want to place a pillow filled with buckwheat or rice on your chest. The weight of the pillow often helps to signal the body to relax and often will gently release any tension that you may be holding in your chest.
  - You will also get a similar response by placing a blanket or shawl over your torso. This is especially relaxing and comforting if the room is chilly, you are tired or jet lagged.
- Keeping your head on the floor, gently tuck your chin into collarbone to elongate the spine. This is a lovely way to practice *Jalandara Bandha*—the chin lock with the weight of your head fully supported by the floor.

If your neck is injury free and it feels good, you may also choose to lift your head UP off the floor on an inhale. As you pause, tuck your chin to your chest, then exhale and slowly release your head to the floor. Always be mindful that you are NOT putting additional strain on the neck or shoulder area.

- Keeping your head on the floor, slowly turn your head side to side. You may choose to inhale, then exhale as you gently rotate to the right, then inhale back to center and exhale as you gently turn to the left. Inhale back to the center and repeat several times until the neck and shoulders soften and relax.

Another neck variation is to turn your head to the right and stay there, breathing gently for anywhere from three to 25-plus breaths. As your body relaxes and releases you'll feel your eyes, face and jaw muscles softening. Eventually your ear may be resting totally on the floor. Be sure to spend equal time on each side and use your inhales and exhales to gently guide you.

All these variations are about releasing tension, so again, be very aware of using your breath to ease in and out of each posture.

- Bring both legs together and center them straight up the wall.
- On your next exhale, open your legs wide until they form the letter "V "against the wall.
  - This may be easier to do if you have socks on because the heels and the weight of your feet will guide your legs as you rest them against the wall. The fabric of your socks will not only protect your heels, but keep your feet warm and accelerate the "slide down the wall."
- Arms may be resting on the floor, palms facing up or down. You may also want to experiment with keeping your hands on your tummy and doing belly breathing. Or you may want to rest your hands on the insides of your thighs, palms facing down, gently breathing into any points of tension and feeling the legs slide further down the wall.

As you do this posture, feel the wall totally supporting the weight of your legs and just breathe. When you are ready to come out of this **"V"** posture, inhale as you gently use your hands on the outside of your knees to gently guide your legs back to center.

"L-O-V-E"

Another fun variation and great breathing stretch is to use your legs up the wall to spell **"L-O-V-E"**. Start in your classical *Viparita Karani* position with your legs straight up the wall.

- Take a few deep inhales and exhales making sure that you are completely comfortable and relaxed. On your next exhale, slowly release your right leg and let it slide down the wall toward the floor. Your right leg will be forming the bottom of the letter **"L"**, and may or may not be resting along the floor. It doesn't matter.
- If there is any tightness or tension in the inner right thigh, you may find that placing the palm of your right hand on your inner thigh will start to soften and release your inner leg muscles.

- Continue gently breathing as your leg gently and slowly begins to move down the wall towards the floor.
  - Remember it is NOT a contest and there is no prize for injuring yourself. So relax and let your breath and gravity do all the work.
- When you are ready to come out of the posture, place your right hand on the outside of your right thigh or the outside of your right knee. Gently guide your leg back up the wall.
  - Repeat the above instructions using your LEFT leg.

After you have done both sides, on an inhale bring both legs back to center so that both legs are resting on the wall.

- On your next exhale slowly bring the soles of your feet together and slide your feet down the wall toward your groin. The outer edges of your feet will be resting on the wall, with your baby toes touching the wall and your heels pressed together sliding down towards your groin. The soles of your feet may or may not be touching. It doesn't matter. The most important element is that you are totally relaxed and comfortable. Your legs will be making the shape of the letter **"O"**.
- Be very mindful of any ankle or knee discomfort and back off slowly. If this feels comfortable, you may want to gently place your hands on the insides of your knees and slowly press your knees towards the wall. Breathe into the inner thighs and any points of tension. Be sure to pay extra attention to the knees. Never press to the point of discomfort or pain. All these postures are meant to be pleasurable.
- If it feels good, you may also want to elongate the spine, by keeping your head on the floor, simply inhale deeply then as you exhale tuck your chin towards your collarbone. Be sure to keep your head ON the floor and continue breathing evenly until you are ready to release the posture. Always use your breath to move your body.

Again, only go as far as feels comfortable. This is NOT a contest and your "O" may not look like a perfect "O". The intention is to gently use your breath and the wall to open up the body.

- Be sure to release your letter "O" by gently bending your knees, placing your heels on the wall and sliding your legs back up the wall into the original *Viparita Karani* position.

Remember at any time, if you've had enough, do not hesitate to stop. Any of these variations can be held for a little as 15-30 seconds to 3-5 minutes. If you listen to your body, you will do exactly what is right for you today.

- The letter **"V"** is the repeat of the variation above. Again, it is easier to do if you have socks on. Simply open your legs and let your breath and gravity slide your heels down the wall until your legs form the letter "V". Be sure to ease in and out of this posture. Stay here for as long as feels comfortable.
- For the letter **"E"** you may want to do the classic "tree pose", or make something up. If you are doing "tree pose", simply slide your right foot down the wall until it is resting on the inside of your left thigh. If this is too much, you may rest your right foot just below your right knee along the calf muscle. Be sure to do the other side and always use the breath to move the body.

If you have had knee surgery or experienced knee injuries, please listen very carefully to your knee joint. The following postures are extremely therapeutic if done properly with healthy knee joints. Always use the breath to move the body and back off if you are experiencing ANY pain or severe discomfort.

Knee Squeeze

- Bring both legs back to center resting straight up on the wall.
- To do a knee squeeze, begin by gently bending your leg and bringing your knee toward you.
- You may wrap your hands under or over the knee cap in order to protect and keep the knee joint stable.
- Experiment with gently moving your leg directly over your chest or keeping it to the outside of the rib cage.
- Direct the knee cap towards the underarm.
- Continue inhaling and exhaling as you squeeze and release the knee towards you. This will give your internal organs and gentle massage and help to keep your hip, knee, and ankle joints lubricated.
- Be sure to do both sides. And notice if one side if easier than the other side.

Side Twists

Side twists can be done several different ways. Have fun and be sure to experiment. Remember to do both sides and notice if the postures are more relaxing with your eyes open or closed.

- Start by bending both knees toward the center of your body over your chest area, and then exhale as you gently drop both knees to the right. You can stay here breathing rhythmically (elongating your inhales and exhales, keeping your eyes soft), or choose to inhale to center then drop both knees to the left.
- If your neck is injury free you may want to coordinate your twist by rotating your head in the *opposite* direction of your knees.
- You may choose to lift your knees a few inches up off the floor and hold as you inhale and exhale.
- Sometimes it feels great to extend both legs straight out to the side resting on the floor.
- Be sure to do both sides and feel free to make up variations that work for you. The wall and the floor will offer complete support.

Climbing the Wall

Climbing the Wall is encouraged **only** if your neck and shoulders are injury free. This is also a wonderful supportive way to work into a free-standing shoulder stand.

- Make sure that you are barefoot, as you start to literally walk your feet up the wall.
- Place your hands on your lower back, fingers facing upwards to support torso.
- Legs may be bent with feet flat against the wall and knees bent. Or you may choose to play with legs up the wall with your heels against the wall or feet flat on the wall.
- You may notice a bit of constriction as the chin is pressed into the collarbone (*Jalandhara Bandha*), be sure to keep the breath steady and even.
- If at any point you experience any discomfort, slowly lower your buttocks to the floor and do a gentle knee hug or squeeze to release any tension in the lower back.
- Only stay up for as long as is comfortable.

Pelvic Tilt

This Pelvic Tilt is also called the *Bundha* Tuck or Reclined *Uddyiana Bandha*. Begin with your legs straight up the wall in the classic *Viparita Karani* position. Heels are resting on the wall and your hands may be placed on your belly or along side your body.

- Gently pull your belly button towards your spine as you press your lower back to the floor.
- Keep breathing. You may add the following *bandhas* or simply exhale and release the belly area.

You may want to experiment with adding *Mulabandha* (The Root Lock), by doing several "Kegels" and then engage *Jalandhara Bandha* (the Chin Lock) by tilting your chin into your collarbone. Breathe and smile, releasing any tension that you may be holding in your face or jaw. When you are ready to release, exhale slowly as you relax the chin away from the collarbone, soften the belly and let the entire pelvic bowl relax.

As with all these postures, please take an extra breath or two before moving into another posture or going onto another activity. I like to call *Viparita Karani* "the cure whatever ails you posture." All of these postures will help you to slow down and move in a more mindful manner. They will also assist you in being present for the next moment.

Note: *Do not do these postures if you have any serious neck or shoulder issues. If at any time you experience any sharp and/or intense pain or constriction, please exhale and move slowly out of the posture. Yoga is not about creating more stress in your life!*

Supine Meditation Pose

Supine Meditation Pose can be with your legs up the wall, simply stretch your arms out in front of you, palms touching, then place your right wrist on top of your left wrist, and turn your hands so that your palms are facing each other, thumbs facing down.

Scoop your licorice rope arms toward you by bending the elbows making a small circle as you bring your interlaced hands toward you and rest them between your breasts. This is a wonderful, nurturing hand mudra and may also be done seated or lying in bed. It is especially soothing if you have insomnia.

Be sure to do the other side, reversing the sequence by placing the left wrist on top of the right wrist. Roll the hands under until the palms touch and the fingers can interlace. Then slowly scoop the hands under and towards you, resting them at your heart center.

When you coordinate this posture with your breathing, it becomes extremely meditative. The weight of your arms will gently press on your chest, especially the heart area, and you may experience a very warm feeling of peace, love, and joy.

#3. The Hassock Asana

This variation is recommended when *Legs Up the Wall* is just too much today, or there is not a clear wall or door in sight. Maybe you need a break between TV commercials and the hassock is just sitting there. Or you are walking through the living room and the hassock is there waiting for you!

- Lie down on the floor next to it and swing your legs up onto it so that your calf muscles are supported by the top of the hassock. It may feel more comfortable to have your legs and knees separated. Experiment gently and see what works for you.
- Be sure that your back is comfortable on the floor, preferably on a carpet or padded surface. Your buttocks may be touching the base of the hassock or several inches away.
- Experiment with finding a comfortable body position. Make sure that your breath is smooth, your face is soft and your jaw is unclenched. The easiest way to relax the entire face is to smile.
- Arms may be at your side, palms facing up or down, or you may choose to place both hands on your belly or between your breasts at your heart center.
- For a deeper meditative *asana*, continue breathing, extending the inhales to match the exhales.
- When it is time to come out of the posture, you may choose to bring your knees up into your chest for a knee hug or squeeze. Then slowly roll onto your side, if possible take a few deep breaths before slowly coming back to a seated position.
- Always make sure that your head is the last part of your body to come up.

Take a few deep breathes to feel centered before going onto your next activity.

༠ᢙᢙᢣ

#4. A Classic Meditation Posture

- Sit on the floor with your back against the wall. Legs should be relaxed, straight out in front of you, slightly apart or comfortably cross-legged. If you are sitting in a chair or in bed, just make sure you have a firm surface to support your back.
- Take a deep inhale as you press your back against the wall.
- Exhale as you feel your shoulders pull down away from the ears.
- Continue inhaling and exhaling, gently and softly elongating each inhale and exhale.
  - Feel any bits of tension melting down into the floor.
  - You may choose to keep your eyes open, closed or half way open gazing at the tip of your nose, your fingers or your toes. Keep your eyes soft.
- Be aware of any tension being held anywhere on your face. Release and relax your upper jaw, lower jaw, and tongue. Feel your mouth softly smiling as your face relaxes.
  - If there is any discomfort in breathing through your nose, be sure to open your mouth and continue to be aware of your inhales and exhales.
- You may choose to tuck your chin into your collar bone using the chin lock. (See *Jalandhara Bandha* in the *Bandha* section).
- Continue breathing, listen to your breath rolling in and out. Stay here as long as you choose. When it is time to release the posture, you may choose to hold your hands in prayer position between your breasts and say a prayer, mantra, or simply kiss your fingertips and thank yourself for being here today.

If you choose to, you may add words (*mantras*) or images (visualizations) to your inhales and exhales. (See the Inhale-Pause-Exhale exercise in the *Pranayama*: Breath Control section, and the *Savasana*: Rest & Relaxation section for more ideas.)

#5. *Asana* Practice 24/7
Weight Management

Many people claim that they have no time to practice yoga or take a class. What they don't realize is that our daily living presents us with constant opportunities to practice yoga. There is nothing in the literature that suggests that one is only practicing yoga while in a yoga studio with specific postures on a special mat.

You may practice yoga anytime and anywhere for as little as a few seconds! In less than a minute you can change how you are feeling by just pausing and taking several deep breaths. When you begin practicing, you will begin to tune into your physical, mental and spiritual body. Just by slowing down and breathing, you will be able to clear the static from your mind and begin to see and feel your reality.

When you name where you are feeling your stress and what it is attached to, you'll have the knowledge to deal with it. This doesn't necessarily mean that you will be able to *cure* whatever ails you, or fix whatever is bothering you in the moment, but you **will** have more internal power to create more space to simply listen. By breathing and noticing where the tension is in your body, you will be able to name it, breathe, and listen to what your body needs in that moment. Maybe you need a walk, a talk with a good friend, a journal session, *legs up the wall,* a nap, or even a few moments to sit and cry. You will find the more you do this practice, the more *in tune* you will be with your reality, and the better able you will be to deal with anything that comes your way.

Try it right now!

- Sit up as straight as you can.
- Relax your facial muscles by smiling gently and unclenching the upper and the lower jaw. Gently tuck your chin towards you collar bone (*Jalandhara bandha*).
- Engage your core muscles by lifting the pelvic floor (*Mulabandha*) and pulling the belly button towards your spine (*Uddiyana bandha*).
- Now slowly take a very deep breath, pause and then let it out as slowly as you can.

How do you feel?

Begin to experiment by incorporating any or all of these basic techniques into your everyday activities. You may practice yoga breathing while sitting in front of the computer, waiting in line, standing in the kitchen chopping vegetables or washing dishes. Begin to find opportunities to add a little more conscious breathing, core lifts, gazing points, rest and relaxation into your daily life.

This is where one runs into that fuzzy line of: *Yoga doesn't get your heart rate up high enough to lose weight, so it really isn't exercise or a good weight management tool.* My personal experience in more than 40 years of practicing this yoga is that it is a priceless practice for weight management. The key is the breath. When I am truly breathing with my entire body and mind, I cannot stuff my face. I cannot gain weight in the moment. *It is only when I am not paying attention,* when I am stressed and not tuning into my breath, that I do something that does not support my health, wealth or happiness. That's when I *fall off the wagon.*

But the good news is that the more I do this practice, especially the breath work, the more my life works. I am better able to make healthy choices. It's a practice. And I am not 100% perfect. Or even close. But I can tell you, the older I get the more this works; and frankly, I don't know any investment that is better than taking care of the one life that you have—right now. Enjoy your next breath. And extra credit if you are smiling!

Questions to Ask Myself

Am I sitting comfortably right now?

Is my breath connected to my body, or am I out of touch with my body thinking about something else?

Where am I right now?

Am I truly in this body of mine?

What can I let go of right now?

Asana is a steady

comfortable posture.

~ Patanjali

This is the Foundation!

Inhale

Pause

Exhale

Pause

Inhale

Pause

Exhale

Pause

Inhale

Pause

Exhale

Pause

Inhale

Pause

Exhale

... **Recharge** ...

rest relax restore revitalize recharge rejuvenate rehabilitate renovate reinvent renew regenerate revive restore refresh release rest relax restore revitalize recharge rejuvenate rehabilitate renovate rest relax restore revitalize recharge rejuvenate rehabilitate renovate reinvent renew regenerate revive restore refresh release rest relax restore revitalize recharge rejuvenate rehabilitate renovate rest relax restore revitalize recharge rejuvenate rehabilitate renovate reinvent

... **Rest & Relaxation** ...

rest relax restore revitalize recharge rejuvenate rehabilitate renovate reinvent renew regenerate revive restore refresh release rest relax restore revitalize recharge rejuvenate rehabilitate renovate rest relax restore revitalize recharge rejuvenate rehabilitate renovate reinvent renew regenerate revive restore refresh release rest relax restore revitalize recharge rejuvenate rehabilitate renovate rest relax restore revitalize recharge rejuvenate rehabilitate renovate reinvent

... **Just Breathe** ...

Chapter 5

Savasana

Rest & Relaxation: Recharging Your Batteries

Questions I've Been Asked

"Why do we always have to do relaxation (savasana) at the end of a yoga pratice?"

Practicing relaxation at the end of a yoga session is considered the icing on the cake. *Savasana* literally translates into *corpse pose,* which is sometimes misleading because you are still breathing! More often, you will hear *savasana* referred to as the **relaxation posture.** After a yoga practice of using the breath to move and stretch your body and your mind, it's ideal to take a few minutes to just pause and let everything come into alignment. The goal is to float in a state of total repose, but not to fall asleep. If you fall asleep, don't worry about it. You obviously need to sleep. I've been known to wake myself up at home or in class by snoring!

"What is the difference between rest and relaxation? Aren't they the same thing?"

Yes and no. Rest implies keeping physically still as in the cessation of work, exertion or activity. It is also closely related to sleep. Relaxation is a more conscious state of awareness usually involving an activity. We often use these words inter-changeably as in experiencing a *relaxing nap,* or a *restful meal.* Rest and relaxation are very subjective. An activity that used to be relaxing may now be stressful, or resting may always be challenging because of all the things on your to-do list.

It is important to remember that the amount of rest we need is dependent on many variables, some things are in our control, and some are out of our control. Factors such as age, health, illness, medications, hormonal levels, travel, season of the year, stress levels, or mental health will affect our rest and sleep patterns. Relaxation is also very individualized. Gardening may totally relax one person, whereas another person prefers to relax by knitting, rock climbing or stock car racing. The more you tune in and fulfill your individual rest and relaxation needs the easier it will be to create and maintain your health.

"I don't have time to rest or relax, not even five minutes, so forget it."

The irony of actually taking five minutes to slow down, relax and rest, is that you will be able to recharge your batteries and actually become more focused, efficient and effective. Many of us are bumblebees, constantly buzzing from one activity to another, or we feel guilty if we just stop for one minute and watch a bird in flight. We are also products of our culture, which rewards us for constantly being busy and producing something tangible, marketable or profitable.

Consciously unplugging for five minutes—to stretch, walk to the bathroom, brush and floss your teeth—is basically so simple and cost effective that you will be surprised at the results.

Find three minutes to walk over to a window and look outside. Take one minute to do some neck rolls, shoulder shrugs or clock eyes (*see Drishti*). Take thirty seconds to stick your tongue out and make a funny face. It doesn't take much to relax. And the return on investment is priceless.

"Why do I have such a hard time resting and relaxing?"

What happens when you hear the words: *relax, take it easy, have a rest, take a break, put your feet up, unwind, take a deep breath, calm down, chill, slow down, loosen up* or *lighten up?*

Is there a part of your mind that says resting and relaxation is a waste of time; that taking a nap is only beneficial for babies and the elderly? Or that resting is only necessary when you are sick or recovering from an injury or a surgery? The body and the mind are continually bombarded with all kinds of stress, seven days a week, 365 days a year. It is often difficult to even schedule predictable relaxation times on a daily basis. It has become increasingly difficult to unplug and that is why practicing yoga techniques can be so beneficial for relaxing and recharging physically, mentally and emotionally.

"Why am so tired when I'm doing an activity I know I should do?"

Sometimes when we are doing something we really don't want to do, it is exhausting. I am curious about what activity you are doing and who told you that you *should* do it? First look at the activity in question and where the *should* is coming from. When you start being honest with yourself you will be able to differentiate why you are *tired*. Are you tired physically? Mentally? Emotionally? Once the truth emerges you can deal with your reality.

Quite often I know I should practice my yoga postures. I know I will feel so much better, happier and healthier. Yet I start the usual litany of excuses: *too tired... too busy... too stressed... too injured... too full... I'll do extra tomorrow.* So I have learned to tell myself, *I'll just practice some yoga postures for five minutes.* And sometimes it *is* only for five minutes, but then sometimes I'm still doing my *asana* practice one hour later. I never know how long those few minutes will actually become, until I start. But I am learning to trust my body-mind to make that decision for me, without beating myself up because I didn't practice for exactly the 1.5 hours blocked out in my appointment book.

"I am always tired and everyone, including my physician, says that I need to relax more. I am really tired of everyone telling me to relax."

Sometimes looking truthfully at ourselves is not a very pleasant task. So we drink another cup of coffee, find a candy bar, a cigarette, a pill, keep working, or see how much we can pile on our plate, literally or figuratively. Or maybe we hardly do anything, why bother to move at all? Maybe your tiredness is working for you. Maybe it gets you off the hook for doing something that needs to be done in your home, at work, or in your family/social life.

Your job is to find out what works for you. Tear off the band-aids and start examining the sore points in your life. Getting to the heart of anything involves a dialog. Start communicating with yourself. Why are you tired? Are certain activities draining you? Is there anything that re-charges your batteries? What is your favorite form of relaxation? I am not talking about nuclear physics here—my total R&R is lying in bed with a great novel, a box of chocolates and a cup of tea! I don't do this every day, but it is one of my personal prescriptions for total bliss. Your job is to find what works for YOU. The choice is always yours.

"I've been overweight and underweight for the past twenty years, and I am tired of feeling like a yo-yo. Now I'm pleasantly plump and miserable. Why can't I get to where I want to be?"

When your body weight is getting in the way of your real life goals, mission, vision and passions, you are out of balance. Weight management is finding your equilibrium between energy in and energy out. And since we are all aging as we speak, everything is constantly changing, hence the continual challenge of connecting with our core self and re-calibrating the scales.

There is a very special balance point for each of us in weight, nutrition, activities, energy, relationships, work, play and recreation. That is why rest and relaxation are so important for the body and the mind. It gives you a chance to catch up with yourself, catch your breath, tune in and figure out what's next. One of the best gifts that you can give yourself is time for rest and relaxation.

I've noticed that sometimes it is hard to *turn the page* in our lives, and get into the next chapter. The more time I take to rest and relax, the happier I am. There is a peace that comes with slowing down so that you can actually hear your true self think. The dialog is priceless and the bottom line is that no one is going to do it for you, it's your life—find it and live it.

"My spouse always takes care of himself first. I am always doing everything for everyone. Then I have no time or energy for myself."

No one but you can make your life a priority. Individuals who are chronically tired, fatigued, overworked, over-stressed, depressed, dealing with eating issues, etc., are usually giving away their energy and not recharging their batteries as they go about their daily activities.

Balanced individuals notice when their *gas tank* is getting low and know exactly how to fill their body and their minds with premium nutrients in the form of breathing, movement, resting, relaxing, eating, drinking water and other recharging activities.

The key is finding out what works for you and doing it consistently, so that you are creating healthy habits. Only you know exactly what you need to do and what works for you! Instead of getting irritated with your spouse, notice what s/he does to recharge. Before doing something for someone else, take a deep breath, and pause. Ask yourself: *Do I really need to do this? If so, does it have to be done right now, this very instant? Can it wait? Am I doing this for them or for me? Will I get mad if I don't get an acknowledgment or recognition for this task?* (Sometimes in the waiting, the task takes care of itself!)

Please note that we all have different styles of working, especially chores. I like to multi-task because it feels efficient. I'll throw in a load of laundry before eating dinner, and then hang it up after dinner. My spouse waits until his laundry basket is overflowing, and then does several loads which takes all morning. We each think the other is inefficient.

There is no easy answer on how to best take care of yourself and your loved ones. Living life, especially with spouses, family and friends is an art and a challenge. I always try to remember the airline safety rule of putting your own oxygen mask on before helping and assisting those around you. Easier said than done; however, there is wisdom in taking care of yourself so that you are fully present to be with the people who need and want you.

"I seem to call in sick once a month and spend a day in bed, reading, eating, sleeping and writing in my journal. I love these days, but I feel guilty pretending that I am sick. How can I get out of this lying?"

I do the same thing. Except I don't call in sick! I actually schedule a day of rest at least once or twice a month. I am flexible about it. If I have an opportunity to do something else that I really want to do—I'll reschedule my day *off*. Just tell people that you have other plans that day, and then take that day for yourself!

Why not make sure you have everything you need the night before —good food, books, relaxing magazines, clean sheets, bubble bath— and go for it! You choose the perimeters for communicating with the outside world including family and/or house mates. Maybe you won't read the news, watch TV, answer the phone, check email or pick up the mail. Or maybe you will. The only thing that matters is that you choose and honor your boundaries.

You'll be surprised how honestly staying in your pajamas or bath-robe one day a month without the guilt of deceit is incredibly empow-ering, enlightening and divinely relaxing. I call them my *vegetable days* or *snow days,* it's an unexpected bonus day, except mine are planned, guilt free and the benefits are priceless!

"My best friend dropped more than 100 pounds this past year and now she is a bundle of energy, walking every day, going back to school, and is so much happier. I am so jealous. I don't even want to be around her."

The good news is that when you start working on your goals in any way, shape or form, and living on purpose, your life will change. One does not suddenly become unbalanced overnight unless you have ex-perienced a deep trauma. Over-weight, under-weight, and all the eat-ing issues in between are rooted in reality. If you really want to change, you have to start examining what is working, and what is not working in your life. It is often hard work, but it is so rewarding, because as your best friend will tell you, one thing leads to another. It's all connected.

If you practice examining yourself with kindness and compassion, you will experience the priceless gift of self-love. Friends can be incred-ibly inspiring and supportive. Ask your friend how she got started on her quest and how she keeps going when things get rough or challeng-ing. Everyone loves to tell their story and give advice. Remember you have to start somewhere, and the best place to begin is exactly where you are.

"I've tried for so many years to do that Positive Thinking thing— think it, believe it, and it will happen. Well, I am still waiting. Nothing good has happened in my life. Yet it seems to work for other people. What am I doing wrong?"

First you have to tell the truth. We sabotage ourselves all the time and then blame our genes, stress, the weather, our mother-in-law, our allergies, our astrological sign, or whatever we can latch onto for something not working.

So what do YOU want and what are you willing to commit toward obtaining that goal? Until your behaviors start moving toward what you want, you can sit chanting positive affirmations until the cows come home. Nothing is going to happen.

We do not live in vacuums. We live in a very juicy, messy and lively world full of controversy, contradictions and challenges. Our job is to continually seek balance and harmony by making adjustments on an as-needed basis in order to survive and thrive. And that goes full circle back to telling the truth. This means dealing with your reality right now this very moment and moving forward. That is the essence of positive thinking and actualization.

When driving a car, riding a bicycle or piloting a jet, one has to keep making adjustments. It's healthy to set goals and leave enough wiggle room to actualize them. When you set clear intentions and your behavior moves toward those goals, doors will open. Positive thinking is all about actually creating movement, and that includes the internal movement of visualizing what you need and want. There is a fine balance between visualizing and actualizing.

It might be helpful to do some of the breathing exercises in the first chapter on *Pranayama*. See if you can inhale, pause, and exhale your needs and wants. See if you can actually say it out loud. What happened? Do your needs and wants ring true for you? The negative is just as important as the positive. And that is why *positive thinking* by itself usually doesn't work. You need to address both sides of the coin.

"Isn't rest and relaxation sort of over-rated? I mean when you die you can sleep forever, so shouldn't we try to cram everything into this lifetime?"

Do not underestimate or trivialize how important rest and relaxation are in finding and maintaining health, equanimity and tranquility. Many studies have shown that lack of sleep, rest and relaxation are often contributors to increased stress-related diseases, disorders and strained relationships. There is no evidence that everyone absolutely needs eight hours of sleep, or that it is necessary to take a nap once a day. Everyone has different physical sleep and rest needs depending on their age and lifestyle. The most important factor is to be willing to observe what works for you and be willing to make the changes you need to give yourself sufficient rest and relaxation. And yes when you die, you may be able to sleep forever; in the meantime why not enjoy and savor as much of life as you can without over-stuffing each day.

"What is the difference between relaxation, meditation, positive affirmations, imagery, visualization, hypnosis, and progressive relaxation techniques?"

We often use the words relaxation, meditation, positive affirmations, imagery, visualization, hypnosis and progressive relaxation techniques interchangeably. Sometimes I will be explaining visualization techniques in class and someone will say: *Oh that's what I do when I meditate.* Or someone will say: *I can't meditate,* but when they describe their relaxation practice it sounds exactly like a description of meditation!

There are many schools of thought, philosophies and practices surrounding all of these techniques. You could approach the task as a chef, looking for the best recipes to try, then experiment and make your own. And as in trying different yoga classes and activities, you may find something that works for you. Many people have found a system or technique that works for them and have practiced the same routine for years; others have buzzed around trying different techniques over the years. So enjoy the journey.

Relaxation is a conscious activity that is a positive experience for the practitioner.

Meditation involves a type of contemplation. Techniques vary depending on the school of thought. Some meditation techniques are based on repeating a mantra, reciting a prayer, focusing on a candle or a photograph of a holy teacher, or breathing mindfully. Some practices encourage just sitting or walking. Some people state that their favorite activity such as running, rowing or dancing is their practice of meditation. (Many activities, when done mindfully, are by definition a meditation.)

Positive affirmations usually involve some combination of reading, writing, and often repeating phrases or sentences out loud, such as: *Every day I am getting healthier and healthier. My tumor is shrinking. I am filled with light and energy. My life is working better than I ever could have expected. Thank you for bringing so much wealth into my life.*

Imagery is forming pictures and/or images in your mind. This powerful tool is often used in moving from disease to health. It can also take the form of putting pictures or photographs of what you need and want where you will see them every day.

Visualization is currently a more popular and familiar term than imagery. Visualization involves creating images in your mind. If you have ever daydreamed or fantasized you are practicing visualization. It is often combined with positive affirmations and pictures, because it reinforces the image of what you need and want.

Hypnosis is a state that resembles sleep, however the person is in a semi-conscious state. This technique usually involves one person instructing the other person with the power of suggestion, or it can be self-induced. Hypnosis is often used as a therapeutic tool in smoking cessation, weight-loss programs, Post-Traumatic Stress Disorder (PTSD) and other trauma or stress-related situations.

Progressive relaxation techniques are a set of instructions on how to use your breath to slowly relax each muscle group in your body. These directions are often set to music or the sounds of nature—like birds chirping, streams running or ocean waves. The goal is to quiet the body, so that it can rest, heal and rejuvenate.

It is important to note that one does not need to lie down on the floor with a pre-recorded DVD or CD, progressive relaxation often happens when making love, taking a walk in the forest or by the ocean, and can even be done in 30 seconds of just tensing the jaw and then yawning. However, it is really a lovely experience if you can take 30 minutes of more to do a complete body scan relaxation sequence.

Note: *You will find all these techniques in the next section.*

Rest & Relaxation Techniques for Stress & Weight Management

#1. Practicing Savasana:
Melting Chocolate on a Hot Summer Day

Although *Savasana* literally translates as the *corpse posture,* it is considered an active meditation posture. The challenge is to totally let go of your physical body as it sinks into a state of deep relaxation, without falling asleep! If you do fall asleep, don't worry about it, you obviously need to sleep. If you are afraid that you will fall asleep and you need to be somewhere at a certain time, then set an alarm to remind you of your next appointment. If your mind wanders as you relax into *savasana,* just let your thoughts float in and out like clouds. The more you practice and experience *savasana,* the more familiar and easier it will become.

The directions here are for lying down on your back, however if that is too uncomfortable for whatever reason, please make the necessary adjustments. You may want to experiment by lying on your side, supported by pillows under your neck or between your knees.

Sometimes it is more comfortable to lie down on your back in a reclining cobbler's pose with the soles of your feet together and your knees out to the side, with your legs making the shape of a diamond. If your knees feel unsupported be sure to put a pillow or a folded blanket under each knee.

Another relaxing variation is to lie on your back with a firm pillow or rolled blanket under your knees. Your knees may be together or separated. You may also choose to practice *savasana* in a recliner chair at home or as a passenger in a car or airplane seat. Whatever position you choose make sure that you are able to safely let your entire body find a fully supported and comfortable resting position.

Savasana is usually easier to access when your clothes are non-binding. If you are wearing a tight belt, scarf or a neck tie make sure that it is loosened, so that your breathing is not constricted. It is also wise to make sure that your body stays warm, by wearing an extra sweatshirt, sweater, or wrapping up in a shawl or a blanket. Sometimes just the gentle weight of a blanket over your body will signal the body/mind that it is time to release any tension. For additional relaxation, you may want to wear socks to keep your feet warm and place a washcloth, hand towel, or an eye-bag over your eyes. Over time you will be able to develop rituals that will signal your body that it is time to let go and relax.

Remember throughout the sequence, you may choose to come out of *savasana* at any time. You also may want to lock the door, add an extra blanket, play music, or do whatever you need to do to keep yourself safe and comfortable.

As you start to tune in to your body, you will notice that it does respond to signals and rituals. Notice what happens tonight when you get into bed and pull the covers up and over your body. Usually we wiggle around a bit, rearranging the pillow, the sheets and blankets until we create a bit of a nest, signaling the body that it is OK to let go—to sleep!

Note: *If you are wearing glasses, take them off and place them in a safe place. If you are wearing contacts, make sure that it is OK to close your eyes for awhile—you may want to remove them; especially if there is a chance you may fall asleep.*

- Lie down on your back or whatever position is most comfortable.
- Close your eyes.
- Be aware of your breathing; just notice your inhales and your exhales.
- Make any adjustments to your body, clothes, blankets or pillows to make sure that you are feeling warm and comfortable before you go any further.
- Feel your body slowly sinking into the floor, bed or chair.
- Let out a really big sigh. You may even want to do several sighs.
- Shake out your arms and legs.
- Relax your arms at your sides, palms facing up.
- On an inhale, squeeze your buttocks together and on an exhale release your buttocks.
- With your head still on the floor, bed or upright in a chair, turn your head side to side, releasing any tension in the neck and upper shoulders. Bring your head back to center, drop the chin down towards your collarbone, then release, and let your head find its natural center.

- Inhale as you squeeze all the muscles in your face making a prune or raisin face, hold this for a few seconds squeezing as tightly as you can, then exhale slowly, releasing all the tension in your face.
- You may feel yourself yawning. Just take your time.
- Relax the eyes and let them roll gently back into their sockets.
- Let a soft smile settle on your lips as you relax the upper jaw and the lower jaw.
- Let the tongue relax.
- Feel the tension in your body melt into the floor, bed or chair.
- Let your inhales and exhales come and go.
- Feel the belly rise and the belly fall.
- Let it all go.

You may want to create an image to further assist your body to relax: *An ice cube or chocolate melting on a hot summer day... Floating on a raft in the middle of a lake or lying under a palm tree on the beach... Standing in a warm shower washing your hair... Sitting in a hot tub... Receiving a massage... Walking into a bakery and smelling cinnamon... Flying in a hot air balloon...*

The combinations are endless and as unique as you are! Stay here as long as you need to or want to. When you are ready to come out of this posture:

- Slowly wiggle your fingers and toes.
- Stretch your arms overhead, as if you were getting up from a long afternoon nap.
- Slowly bring your knees up to your chest or along the sides of your rib cage for a knee squeeze or knee hug.
- You may want to rock side to side, or up and down a few times, or just drop your knees to one side and then slowly to the other for a gentle twist.
- Whatever you choose to do, please do it mindfully and slowly.
- There is absolutely no rush.
- Listen to your body, it will tell you what you need to do.
- When you are ready, roll onto your right or left side.
- Stay curled up on your side for at least three deep inhales and exhales.
- As you slowly come up into a seated position, make sure that your head is the very last part of your body to come up.
- Sit quietly and just enjoy that wonderful feeling of peace and tranquility.

#2. The Body Scan for Releasing Tension

The purpose of this practice is to find the answer to: *Where am I holding tension?*

This body scan involves slowly naming each part of your body as you squeeze and then release it. The first practice involves going through your entire body. The second practice describes how to do mini-body scans when you only have a few minutes.

Please remember that this is a lifetime practice and not a quick fix. It took years for many of us to accumulate tension in various parts of our bodies, and it will take time to tune in and release that tension.

- Find a comfortable position. If you are lying down or in a recliner chair, you may choose to cover your eyes with a lightly scented eye bag, hand towel or wash cloth.
- Close your eyes.
- Take three deep inhales and exhales.
- Very slowly begin the body scan, by starting from the toes and working your way up to the top of your head. Just say to yourself (or have someone read this to you):
  - bring your awareness to your toes…
  - squeeze your toes as tightly as you can, then slowly release your toes…
  - bring your awareness to your feet… now squeeze your feet as tightly as you can…
  - then release your feet and let them rest heavy…

Using the following list as a guide, continue moving up the body. Remember if any part of your body feels extra tight, painful or just blah, you may choose to repeat the name of that part several times, until you feel your body releasing and relaxing even further.

I personally like to begin with my toes; however, you may choose to begin with your head, or change the order of the list. The most important element is to do what works for you *today*. And if you don't have enough time to do the whole sequence, just choose a body part or area that is bothering you right now.

Tension can always be released with a big yawn or simply sticking out your tongue as you stretch your mouth as wide as it will go. Super exaggerate both stretches and you will feel immediate relief!

When going through the entire body, I sometimes start with the right (toes) and then the left (toes) and go back and forth. Sometimes I do right leg, then left leg and slowly move up the body. I've also noticed that I don't always do every single part of my body, or will suddenly be inspired to say *lymph nodes*, so I have learned to just take it as it comes. The true test is how do you feel when you are finished?

Toes
Feet
Ankles
Shins
Calves
Knees
Thighs
Inner Groins
Hips
Reproductive Organs
Intestines
Stomach
Liver
Kidneys
Breasts
Heart
Lungs
Chest
Shoulders
Upper Arms
Elbows
Forearms
Wrists
Hands
Fingers
Neck
Throat
Chin
Mouth
Lips
Tongue
Nose
Nostrils
Eyebrows
Ears
Inner Ears
Eyes
Back of the Eyes
Forehead
Hair
Skull
Back of the Head
Top of the Head

When you get to the crown of your head, take three deep inhales and exhales. Feel your body releasing and relaxing even further.

- Take the next three deep inhales and exhales as slowly as you can—breathe through your toes, feeling the breath move up through your body and then exhale your breathe out through the top of your head.
- Feel your face softening, jaw relaxing and eyes sinking gently into the back of your head.
- Let a soft smile settle onto your face and throughout your body.
- Let your body/mind be your guide. You may fall asleep, or choose to go to a favorite place in your mind's eye—the beach, the mountains, a forest, a beautiful garden, anywhere that gives you instant relaxation. Just linger and enjoy your surroundings.
- You may stay here as long as you choose.
- If you are going to get up and go about your day or evening, please make sure you take your time. If you are lying down, you may choose to do some gentle stretches while still on your back (yawning, stretching your arms overhead, giving yourself a knee squeeze or hug), before you roll onto your side taking a few gentle breaths. Press one hand into the bed or floor as you roll up into a seated position, making sure that your head is the last part of your body to come up.
- Sit quietly and take a few breaths to go inside and sincerely thank your body, mind and spirit for traveling with you.
- Slowly open your eyes and acknowledge that you can take all this good energy with you out into your day or your evening.

Note: *If you are relaxing into a nap or going to sleep, take a moment to shake out your entire body, releasing any kinks or leftover tensions, then totally surrender and enjoy a very peaceful rest.*

Do not do this while driving, operating complicated machinery or at any time where you need to be fully present in the physical dimension.

Mini Scans 24/7

The more you practice this technique, the more familiar you will become with your tension spots. You will be able to do *mini scans* by taking a deep breathe and asking yourself: *Where am I holding tension?* As soon as you name the body part that is tense, you will be able to squeeze and release tension wherever you are. This technique does not require a huge time commitment, short sessions work just as well.

Mini body scans are also good to do before you go to sleep, especially if you are restless and have a lot going on in your mind. Just concentrate on the individual parts of your body that are tense, if you don't want to go through your entire body from head to toes. Sometimes just resting your hands on your belly and slowly breathing in and out will help relax the entire body so that you can release and fall sleep.

Belly Breathing, Moving Up the Body

This is good practice to do before you go to sleep or take a nap. So much of our daily stress can be related to not having good night's sleep. We often mistake fatigue for hunger and then eat, when in fact we need a nap! Be sure to read though this dialog and feel free to modify it to fit your needs today. You can also break it up and use individual elements—you don't need to do the whole thing. For example, place your hand on your belly as you are sitting upright in a chair and breathe in and out. This even works at stop lights or sitting in a traffic jam. It's a wonderful, peaceful and rejuvenating mini meditation.

If you are wearing glasses or contacts, you may choose to take them off and keep them in a safe place near you.

- Lic flat on your back and close your eyes. If you are too uncomfortable on your back, lie on your side. You can do this practice with your feet up the wall, seated in a chair or in bed.
- Shake out your body until your body weight is equally and comfortably resting on the floor, chair, couch or bed.
- Rest your right hand gently on your belly just below your belly button.
- Let your belly rise with each inhale and fall with each exhale.
- Just let your breathe move in and out.
- Feel your body relaxing, and melting into the floor or chair.

Rest here for five to ten breaths, enjoy breathing slowly and gently.

- Now place your left hand above your belly button, keeping the right hand below the belly button.
- Just feel your breath going in and out through your nose.
  - Be sure to open your mouth if you feel any constriction or congestion in your throat, eyes, nose or head.
- After five to ten deep breaths, pick up your right hand and place it between your breasts at your heart center.
- Keep your left hand above your belly button and feel the connection between your breath and your heart. Feel your heart gently beating. Relax the face, unclench the jaw, relax the tongue and feel a soft smile forming on your lips.

Rest here for five to ten breaths, enjoy breathing slowly and gently.

- Now place your left hand gently on your throat, feeling the pulse in your neck. Leave your right hand resting between your breasts.
- Feel the breath moving up and down the highway of your throat.
- Enjoy the sensation of breathing for the next five to ten breaths, then pick up your right hand and gently place it on your forehead.
  - Feel all your winkles and worries just melting away into the ground.
- Leave your left hand on your throat as you feel all the muscles on your face relaxing as your face becomes as soft and smooth.

Continue breathing in and out for five to ten breaths.

- Keeping your eyes closed, slowly release your hands, extend your arms out in front of you with your palms touching.
- Vigorously rub your hands together until they become warm, they may even become hot.
- Gently place your hands over your eyes, creating a *cup* over your eyes—fingers resting gently on the forehead and the heels of your hands resting lightly on your cheeks.
  - Be careful not to exert any pressure on the eyes. If you are wearing contacts, please be extra gentle.
- Feel the warmth penetrating all the muscles in your face.
- Feel your face becoming softer with each inhale and exhale.

After five to ten breaths, slowly lower your arms to your side, palms facing up. And enjoy the next few minutes of bliss. If you are going to continue with your day or evening, take a few moments to visualize everything going smoothly.

- Be sure to take your time, by slowly stretching your arms overhead, bringing your knees into your chest for a knee hug or squeeze before you roll onto your side.
- Then as slowly as you can, take your time to come back to a seated position. Make sure that your head is the last part of your body to come up.
- Be sure to sit up as straight as you can and take a few deep breaths before you move on to your next activity.

⌒◟◞⌒

#3. Guided Relaxation & Visualization

This guided relaxation and visualization was created to recharge your physical, mental, emotional and spiritual batteries. You may want to record it, or find a friend to read it to you. It is best to do this in a quiet place where you will not be interrupted. Please feel free to change the dialog by adding or deleting choice phrases. The most important element is to find words, images, and concepts that work for you today.

To begin this positive relaxation and visualization process, find a comfortable position sitting on a chair or couch or lying down on a recliner, a bed or the floor. Loosen your belt and take off your shoes. If you are wearing glasses, you may want to take them off and put them in a safe place.

If you are lying down, find a comfortable position resting on your back or your side. You may choose to bend your knees to release any stress or tension in the lower back by placing a pillow or blanket under or between your knees.

You may also choose to put your legs up the wall while resting on your back. Wherever you are, do whatever you need to do to **maximize** your physical comfort level. You may put a shawl, blanket or comforter over your body.

The Basic Dialog

For the next ten minutes you will be using your breath to guide your body, mind and spirit into a deeper state of relaxation.

- Begin by shaking out your arms and legs.
- Point and flex your feet.
- Move your head from side to side.

- Release your right ear down toward your right shoulder.
- Next, release your left ear down toward your left shoulder.

Feel the tension from your neck and shoulders melting into the chair or onto the floor.

- Open your mouth as wide as you can until you feel a yawn. Take your time yawning as big and wide and deep as you can.
- Then slowly begin to tune into your breath. Be aware of your inhales and your exhales. Take the next few breaths to just listen to the rise and fall of your chest as you inhale and exhale.
- There is nothing to do, nowhere to go, just listen to your breath. Allow your eyes to gently close.

Give your body permission to totally let go, release and relax.

- Take a deep, deep inhale. Pause. Listen and exhale slowly, sending your breath to any part of your body that needs a little extra tender loving care.
- Feel your body relaxing as it melts into the chair or the floor.
- Take another deep inhale. Pause. And again, send your exhale to any part of your body that still feels tight, tense or tender.

Feel all the tension in your body dissolving and melting away down into the earth.

- Take another deep breath. Pause. As you exhale mentally say the word, *Relax...* (or any word that conjures relaxation for you, *Release, Melt, Let Go, Let It Be...*).

You are now at a deeper, healthier, more relaxed state of awareness.

- Imagine that you are surrounded by soft, warm, clean, fresh air.
- Feel this air circulating around you, and throughout your body, let this wonderful fresh, soft, warm air nurture your body, your mind, and your spirit.
- Visualize yourself somewhere that you love. This place can be real or imaginary. Maybe you are on the beach. Lying on the warm soft sand... looking up at the sky through the palm trees...
- Or hiking along a mountain stream, or lying in a grassy meadow surrounded by wildflowers and birds chirping...
- Or maybe you are rowing on beautiful crystal clear lake... watching a spectacular sunrise... or sunset...

- Maybe you are sitting on a porch sipping lemonade on a warm summer afternoon… Or hanging out in your favorite coffee shop, bookstore or library…
- Take a few breaths to find a quiet, safe and peaceful place.

Feel a sense of relaxation settling into your body.

- Feel your body… heavy… warm… soft.
- Feel your face relaxing as your upper jaw releases from your lower jaw.
- Feel your tongue resting at the back of your mouth.
- Feel a soft smile playing on your lips. As if you know the secret to the universe.
- As you take your next inhale and exhale. Feel your body relaxing.

As you take the next three deep breaths, feel your body relaxing and releasing even deeper…

Inhale/pause/exhale…
Inhale/pause/exhale…
Inhale/pause/exhale.

Continue breathing and just let your body and your mind wander.

- Just observe, let go, release and relax.
- Stay here for as long as you choose to do so.

Remember, when you are ready to return from your journey, take your time coming out very slowly and mindfully.

If you are lying down, you may choose to do some gentle stretches while still on your back (yawning, stretching your arms overhead, giving yourself a knee squeeze or hug). What ever you do, take your time before you roll onto your side taking a few gentle breaths. Press one hand into the bed or floor as you roll up into a seated position, making sure that your head is the last part of your body to come up.

Sit quietly and take a few breaths to go inside yourself and sincerely thank your body, mind and spirit for supporting you.

Slowly open your eyes and smile, knowing that you may take all this good energy with you out into your day or your evening.

∽⊙⤬⊙∼

#4. Creating *Mantras:* Let It Be

A *mantra* is a syllable, word, phrase, image, quote, poem or prayer that is used to focus the mind. The word *mantra* literally translates to *man* (mind) and *tra* (free and deliver). *Mantras* are meant to unite the mind and the body and ultimately create a sense of oneness with the universe.

"What is the best mantra to use?"

Mantras work best when they personally resonate with you. Find a word or image that makes you smile and gives you a sense of peace and relaxation. Remember this *mantra* is only set in stone if you choose it to be. There is nothing in the universe that says that one must keep your *mantra* for a lifetime. Many of us have several *mantras*.

"Does my mantra have to be a sacred word?"

It can be whatever you choose. Sometimes just a phrase of a song, poem or prayer may serve as a wonderful touchstone. Just repeating a word or words that mean something to you can be totally relaxing. Some people use a phrase such as:

One...

Yummmmmm...

Om... or Aum...

All is well...

I am at peace...

Om mani padme om... (*Om the jewel is in the lotus crown.*)

Jesus loves me...

Shalom... Peace... Love... Aloha...

Mary, mother of all...

You are my sunshine...

May all beings be peaceful, may all beings be happy, may all beings be safe, may all beings awaken to the light of their true nature, may all beings be free. (Loving Kindness Meditation)

Our father, who art in heaven...

So-hum (I am that.)

Om Namah Shivaya (The *Panchakshara mantra* with many interpretations including: *I honor the divinity within me.*)

Aum Bhuh Bhuvah Svah Tat Savitur Varenyam Bhargo Devasya Dheemahi Dhiyo Yo nah Prachodayat. (The *Gayatri mantra* with many translations and interpretations, including *Swami Vivekananda's:* "We meditate on the glory of that Being who has produced this universe, may he enlighten our minds.")

Mantras can be used to keep the body, mind and spirit focused all day. Think of an old favorite song that you hear on the radio in the morning and end up humming all day long with a smile on your face. That's a working *mantra!*

"When do I practice saying my mantra?"

Anytime that works for you! You can be organized in a seated meditation position, or incorporate your mantra into your everyday activities. I like to repeat my *mantra* as I am walking the dog, waiting in line, sitting in traffic, washing the dishes, mowing the lawn, or before I go to sleep. Remember that *mantras* can be repeated silently, out loud, sung or chanted. Driving in a car makes a great *mantra* container (the acoustics are almost as good as singing in the shower!) Have fun!

"Do I need prayer beads?"

Prayer beads, bracelets, rosaries or touchstones are totally optional. Just make sure whatever you choose to do is increasing peacefulness and joy, and not a distraction or causing more stress and discomfort.

"My brother has a tattoo of a lotus blossom with the words God is Good on his arm, he says that every time he looks at it, it calms him down. Is that a mantra?"

By my definition, yes! The combination of the image and the words makes a sound—either silently in his head, or he says it out loud. Either way he has his own personal *mantra* that helps him focus.

"Shouldn't you have someone important tell you your mantra? Like in a religious ceremony or something official?"

Mantras do not have to be delivered by a holy person with a ceremony attached. This is a very individual and personal choice. It is also a choice if you choose to share your *mantra*. You probably already have a word or song that personally resonates with you and that has been used before. As long as you are happy with your *mantra*, it really doesn't matter who gave it to you or where you found it.

"I love to listen to chants, are those mantras?"

Personally, I think that any sacred chant or music that puts you into a meditative receptive mood can be considered a *mantra*. By definition, chants are usually short and simple melodies. I know that some scholars, teachers and practitioners would disagree with me; however, the bottom line is, how does chanting make you feel and what chants resonate with you today.

"So it really doesn't matter what word you choose to focus on?"

The most important element of a having a personal *mantra* is that it resonates with you. Someone can give you a beautiful word to chant or focus on, but unless it really rings true for you, it will just be a word. Think of someone you really love. Then say their name out loud. What happened?

Now think of a random name or someone you really are having issues with and say their name out loud. You may notice a very different response. (And you may choose to do one of the breathing techniques in Chapter One to bring some equilibrium into that relationship.)

In the meantime, have fun trying on different *mantras*. See if you can find some words or images that resonate deep within you. Sometimes when I am stuck or moping around, I'll just say to myself: **Chocolate Yoga** or *How can I turn this into a* **Chocolate Yoga** *moment?*, or the classic, *This too shall pass.* Those words totally shift my focus into a happier, healthier and more productive place!

"You make it sound so easy. I really don't know where to start?"

First of all, you already have some answers right now. Write down the titles or words from a few of your favorite songs. Then write or draw some of the images and words that make you smile. You may want to pick up a book of quotes, a book of paintings, look around your house, take a walk, or go to a library or bookstore.

You are surrounded by words and images that nurture you and give you joy. Just think back to happy moments in your life. I have a favorite beach that I haven't been to in years, but usually once a day, I say the name of that beach silently or out loud and feel instantly refreshed and focused. It is a code word for me to create a sense of calming bliss. Even as I say it right now, I can hear the waves, feel the soft balmy air, and see the endless stretch of beach. Your code word can be as simple as saying: *puppies; mocha;* or *smile.* Enjoy the process of exploring. It also helps to have a sense of humor. And remember that it's OK to have several *mantras,* use them for different situations, and to change them as often as you see fit. I like to think of *mantras* as having many supportive friends who are always there for you.

"So how do I use these mantras for rest and relaxation?"

Your *mantra* is available to you 24/7. When you are feeling in need of some rest and relaxation, just repeat your *mantra* silently or out loud. Your *mantra* is a signal to your mind to connect to your body, and in the process you will feel that sense of rest and relaxation. Your *mantra* can serve as a comforter—like a child's favorite blanket or lullaby. It's instant and it's free!

You may choose to add breathing techniques to your *mantra,* but often just a few repetitions of your *mantra* will get you into a healthier frame of mind. Remember that one does not have to sit in a full meditation posture to benefit from mantras. You can use *mantras* throughout your busy day—driving to work or the store, running errands, sweeping the floor, changing diapers, washing dishes, waiting in line, sitting on an airplane—the possibilities are endless.

#5. A Lifetime Meditation Practice for Weight Management

The root of the word *meditation* comes from the Latin *meditatum,* (to ponder). Other definitions of meditation include: *to mull over, contemplate, study, think, ruminate, cogitate,* and my favorite, *to chew on!* The word meditation is also closely related to *mederi* (to heal). If you put these two concepts together, you will be able to create endless opportunities to meditate all day without moving to a cave up in the mountains.

The next time you are resenting doing something, especially chores or an activity that you have to do, turn it into a meditation. Simply say: *This is my* (fill in the blank) *meditation.* It takes the sting out of the pressure of **having** to do something. The benefits are instant relaxation. And if you dream of being able to meditate all day, here is your opportunity!

Begin by turning your chores into mini-mediations. We all have an endless to-do list and often resent the list and/or the pressure. However, I am learning to turn everything into meditation and I feel much more rested, and relaxed. Simple *little* things such as taking a shower, walking the dog, grocery shopping, or doing the laundry can be turned into a meditation.

This also works for activities that you **should** do, simply because you love someone and it means a lot to them (driving your children to their music or soccer practice, making an appointment for your busy spouse, or showing up at a function simply because it is the right thing to do). Or even doing something you know that is **good for you!**

This is my walking meditation. This is my eating vegetables meditation, or *This is my flossing meditation.* I use this one every day on my way to work: *This is my working for the mortgage and my tax contribution for better schools meditation.*

By practicing the *little* and *medium* meditations, you will be building muscle to practice the *bigger* meditations involving more difficult life and death situations. Maybe you have to attend a funeral, deal with a diagnostic test for cancer, or support a spouse who is suddenly out of a job. Try to re-frame these situations into meditations and see what happens:

This is my going to a funeral meditation.

This is my diagnostic tests for cancer meditation.

This is my listening to my spouse (child, mother in law, boss) meditation.

This does not mean you are a doormat by listening; in fact you will notice a very interesting dynamic when you are totally focused and truly listening, the other person will start to absorb your calmness and often work out their situation without any direct input from you. I call this my: *Shut up and listen meditation.*

If at any time you feel emotional pain, it is important to deal with it. You may journal, seek a health professional, or choose to dialog directly with the person who is part of your pain. Please always remember to be honest and speak from the heart. A broken heart is an open heart.

You will find meditation opportunities as you go about your daily activities and you will be able use your life to explore, live and learn. So much of our stress is rooted in the things we *need* to do, the things we *want* to do and the things we think we *should* do.

When you begin to mix all these voices in your head, you will notice that your body gets confused and becomes so disconnected that you truly do not know if you are thirsty, hungry, tired or climbing up the wrong mountain.

By calming the mind with *mantras*, you will be able to hear your inner truth. This is a practice, so give it some time. You may experience instant insights or you may feel as if you are wandering around hopelessly in the dark. If you can slow down and breathe, you will be able to slow down your mind.

Think of all your stressors as snowflakes in one of those globes that you turn upside down, and then sit and watch all the flakes slowly settle down to the ground. Over time you will be able to access this skill and be able to really tune into your truth. **The benefit is that it will help you manage your weight.** You will be able to tune into what you really need and want.

The good news—
Your breath is free and available 24/7.

And ultimately you are making the best investment in your life—your health, wealth, and happiness will grow through this practice.

Questions to Ask Yourself

What is the most relaxing thing that I could do for myself right NOW?

Am I getting enough rest and relaxation in my life?

What word or image gives me peace?

What can I let go of right now?

Yoga-citta-vritti-nirodhah.
(Yoga is the cessation of the
chattering of the mind.)

~ Patanjali

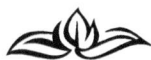

This is the Foundation!

Inhale

Pause

Exhale

Pause

Inhale

Pause

Exhale

Pause

Inhale

Pause

Exhale

Pause

Inhale

Pause

Exhale

... Living ...

Living Chocolate Yoga Living Chocolate Yoga

... Chocolate Yoga ...

Living Chocolate Yoga Living Chocolate Yoga

... Just Breathe ...

Conclusion

Living Chocolate Yoga

Putting It All Together

The Ultimate Chocolate Yoga Meditation

Just how slowly can you savor and enjoy a tiny piece of chocolate melting in your mouth?

Notice how often we swallow, inhale, and rush though all our snacks and meals.

What's the rush?

Whose life is this, anyway?

Why am I in such a hurry?

What will happen if I slow down?

What can I let go of right now?

Note: *This* **Chocolate Yoga** *Meditation is the foundation of Living* **Chocolate Yoga***. The big question is why we can't do this practice 24/7. The answer is simple, we are too busy. And that is OK. By practicing this* **Chocolate Yoga** *meditation, over time you will slowly learn that you can take a deep breath and actually live the life you want to live. This* **Chocolate Yoga** *meditation takes approximately 15–20 minutes.*

Find a comfortable seated position on the floor, chair or couch. You may do this sitting up in bed if you are leaning against something firm.

Place a small piece of chocolate, on a small plate. (If chocolate doesn't work for you—find something sweet like a small raisin, grape or baby carrot.) Place the plate about three feet away from you. Take two to three minutes to just stare at the chocolate. Let your thoughts come and go like clouds on a windy day. Feel your eyes soften and relax. There is nothing to do except mindfully inhale and exhale. Continue to let your thoughts come and go.

It you get stuck on a thought just say, *That's interesting.* Or *I'll deal with that later.* Continue to inhale and exhale as slowly as you can.

After a few minutes, reach out and bring the plate about two feet in front of you. Continue to relax your eyes and see if you can lengthen your inhales and exhales. I usually get very distracted at this point, so if I am alone, I say out loud, *Inhale... pause... exhale.* Just hearing my voice and listening to my breathing helps me focus on the chocolate in front of me.

Your breathing at this point will probably begin to sound like ocean waves going in and out along the shore. If your breath is choppy, or one or both nostrils are stuffy, just breathe as best you can and observe.

After a few minutes move the plate so that it touches your leg or knees. Your chin may be tucked in a bit so that you may continue to gaze comfortably at the chocolate.

After a few more minutes take the piece of chocolate off the plate and place it in your hands, palms facing up. I like to place my right hand on top of my left hand in my lap with the palms facing up. Tuck your chin into your chest and gaze down at the chocolate. Continue breathing as smoothly as you can.

After another minute, slowly pick up the chocolate and take a **tiny** bite. Place the rest of your chocolate back on the plate and close your eyes. Let your hands rest in a comfortable position on your thighs or the middle of your lap. Let the chocolate melt. Just observe the taste sensations and note the inner dialog.

Just observe. Continue breathing and see if you can become engaged with that piece of melting chocolate. Let the chocolate completely melt.

See if you can just sit and breathe and enjoy the afterglow of that piece of chocolate. After a few minutes, slowly open your eyes. Note the remaining piece of chocolate. Notice what you are thinking and feeling. There is nothing to do. Just observe.

What Did You Learn?

- That a tiny piece of chocolate can be as fulfilling as a whole box of chocolates?
- That I can be satiated with less?
- That I don't need to eat an entire burger or meal to feel full?

How can I create more **Chocolate Yoga** moments in my life right now? How can we carry this wonderful feeling of serenity, centeredness, and peacefulness into our everyday life? How can one find joy in our daily tasks? And what does one do about the problems and situations that arise simply because we live in an unpredictable, chaotic and juicy world. This is the challenge. And **Chocolate Yoga** is the answer.

This yoga is not about waving a magic wand and having every thorn in our life disappear. It is about acknowledging everything in our lives and dealing with it as it arises. Stresses will continue to ebb and flow through our life until we die. It is our responsibility to meet and greet our stressors, big and small, and then make conscious healthy decisions do deal with them over time. This includes choosing to ignore, or postpone dealing with a stressor, until the time is right for you.

All this yoga comes from the heart, and that is the ultimate challenge. **Can I live my life from my heart?** It's a lifelong practice, so please lighten up. We tend to *beat ourselves up* over and over again, as we deal with the issues in our life. There comes a time to acknowledge that we are doing the best we can under the circumstances.

And if you can create some healing in feeding your body, mind, and soul, you will begin to notice to following:

1. Stress is here to stay. Deal with it.

2. Diets don't work unless you address your stress issues.

3. Yoga postures are only the tip of the iceberg. Yoga is much deeper. Practicing yoga will help you manage your stress and weight issues for the rest of your life.

4. Health, wealth and happiness are created and nurtured from within.

5. There are many paths up the mountain. Find what works for you. When you get to the top of the mountain… keep climbing.

No one can *tell* you how to live your life. The challenge is to figure out just how to live your life and not only survive, but to thrive. My hope for you is that you found a piece of **Chocolate Yoga** that works for you. That somehow in the midst of all these words that you were able to connect to your body and mind through the spirit of your breath and move toward creating more health, wealth, and happiness in your everyday life.

I sincerely hope that you are finding more ways to appreciate your wonderful body, to mindfully feed and care for it as best you can. I hope you are finding light and opportunities between the big and little stresses in your life. I also hope that you can feel your breath moving you in the right direction. And that your next breath brings you much peace and happiness.

And most of all, I do hope that these yoga gifts of *Pranayama, Bandhas, Drishti, Asanas* and *Savasana* feed and nurture your body, mind, and spirit for a lifetime.

Namaste

Questions to Ask Yourself

*How can I turn this moment into a **Chocolate Yoga** opportunity?*

Am I breathing?

What is the best use of my time right now?

What can I let go of right now?

Welcome to the Rest of Your Life.

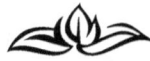

This is the Foundation!

Inhale

Pause

Exhale

Pause

Inhale

Pause

Exhale

Pause

Inhale

Pause

Exhale

Pause

Inhale

Pause

Exhale

Quick Guides for Exercises

Chapter 1: *Pranayama,* **The Breath:**
Connecting the Body & the Mind.
Yoga Breathing Techniques for Stress & Weight Management

1. **Instant Stress Relief 24/7:** Inhale, Pause, Exhale.
2. *Nadi Shodana:* Alternating Nostril Breathing.
3. *Ujjayi* **Breathing:** Close Mouth, Breathe Through the Nose.
4. *Kalapathi* **Breathing:** Rapid Bellows Breathing, Pulling Belly Button Towards the Spine.
5. **Put Your Fork Down:** Take a Deep Inhale, Pause, and Exhale.

Chapter 2: *Bandhas,* **Energy Locks:**
Creating Core Heat.
Increasing Core Energy for Stress & Weight Management

1. *Mulabandha:* Kegel-like Lift 24/7.
2. *Uddiyana Bandha:* Belly Button to the Spine.
3. *Jalandhara Bandha:* Chin to Collarbone.
4. **The Great Lock:** Simultaneously Engage the Above Three *Bandhas.*
5. **Walking Tall:** Stand, Sit or Walk with shoulders rolled back and away from the ears, head erect, facial muscles relaxed, belly button towards the spine, and pelvis tucked.

Chapter 3: *Drishti,* The Gazing Points:
Looking In & Looking Out.
Drishti Techniques for Stress & Weight Management

1. **Clock Hands:** Rotate eyes clockwise and counter-clockwise.

2. **Warm Hands Mini Spa:** Rub your hands together then release over eyes.

3. **Hand Mudras:** Fingers touching to connect to your heart.

4. **The Reality Journal:** May be written or drawn on any medium that works for you. Use it as a way to **dig** down real deep to find the root of your issues. If you are ever stuck writing, just begin listing all the things that you are angry or depressed about, or all the things you are grateful for. Both lists are very interesting. Be curious and explore.

5. **Name that Focus:** Also known as *talking to yourself.* This is a very practical tool for bringing attention and focus to reality. This technique will help you stay grounded in the moment by simply stating what you are doing or thinking in this very moment. Including eating a whole bag of chips!

Chapter 4: *Asanas,* The Postures:
Meditation in Motion.
Body Postures for Stress & Weight Management

1. **Legs Up The Wall:** Find a clear wall space and lying on your back, put your legs up the wall. You may also use a hassock or lying in bed, stack a whole bunch of pillows under your knees, calves and feet.

2. **Variations of Legs Up the Wall:** L-O-V-E and Climbing the Wall.

3. **The Hassock *Asana.***

4. **Classic Meditation Posture.**

5. ***Asana* Practice 24/7 for Weight Management:** Every posture can be turned into an *asana.*

Chapter 5: *Savasana*, Rest and Relaxation: Recharging Your Batteries.
Rest & Relaxation Techniques for Stress & Weight Management

1. **Practicing *Savasana*:** *Melting Chocolate on a Hot Summer Day*

2. **Body Scan for Releasing Tension:** Naming each body part from toes to top of head, mini-scans 24/7, and belly breathing.

3. **Guided Relaxation and Visualization:** Dialog to release physical tension and create emotional support with positive visualization.

4. **Creating Mantras: Let it be!** Choosing words or phrases that create calm, peace and joy within you.

5. **A Lifetime Meditation for Weight Management:** Reframing your chores, tasks and habits as *mini-meditations* to assist you in creating health, wealth and happiness within.

The Ultimate Chocolate Yoga Meditation:

Just how slowly can you savor and enjoy a tiny piece of chocolate melting in your mouth?

Notice how often we swallow, inhale, and rush though all our snacks and meals.

What's the rush?

Whose life is this, anyway?

Why am I in such a hurry?

What will happen if I slow down?

What can I let go of right now?

... Just Breathe ...

inhale – pause – exhale– pause – inhale – pause – exhale– pause
– inhale – pause – exhale – pause – inhale – pause – exhale–
pause – inhale – pause – exhale– pause – inhale – pause –
exhale – pause – inhale – pause – exhale– pause – inhale
– pause – exhale– pause – inhale – pause – exhale – pause –
inhale – pause – exhale– pause – inhale – pause – exhale– pause
– inhale – pause – exhale – pause – inhale – pause – exhale

... Just Breathe ...

inhale – pause – exhale– pause – inhale – pause – exhale– pause
– inhale – pause – exhale – pause – inhale – pause – exhale–
pause – inhale – pause – exhale– pause – inhale – pause –
exhale – pause – inhale – pause – exhale– pause – inhale
– pause – exhale– pause – inhale – pause – exhale – pause –
inhale – pause – exhale– pause – inhale – pause – exhale– pause
– inhale – pause – exhale – pause – inhale – pause – exhale

... Just Breathe ...

About the Author

Margaret Chester has a Masters Degree in Public Health and is a Registered Yoga Teacher. She had always wanted to be a yoga teacher, but thought she couldn't teach until she was skinny and could get her foot behind her head! After years of struggling with her stress and weight issues, she has found a way to survive and thrive by practicing *Chocolate Yoga*. She is currently teaching workshops.

Please visit

ChocolateYoga.com

www.ingramcontent.com/pod-product-compliance
Lightning Source LLC
Chambersburg PA
CBHW072250270326
41930CB00010B/2331